TOBACCO USE PREVENTION MEDIA CAMPAIGNS:
LESSONS LEARNED FROM YOUTH IN NINE COUNTRIES

Sponsored by the Centers for Disease Control and Prevention

Authors

Elizabeth Schar, Marketing Consultant

Karen Gutierrez, Marketing Consultant

Rebecca Murphy-Hoefer, PhD, MPH, Health Communications Specialist, Office on Smoking and Health/CDC

David E. Nelson, MD, MPH, Senior Scientific Advisor, Office on Smoking and Health/CDC

March 2006

Suggested citation: Schar E, Gutierrez K, Murphy-Hoefer R, Nelson DE. *Tobacco Use Prevention Media Campaigns: Lessons Learned from Youth in Nine Countries*. Atlanta: U.S. Department of Health and Human Services, Centers for Disease Control and Prevention, National Center for Chronic Disease Prevention and Health Promotion, Office on Smoking and Health; 2006. Available at www.cdc.gov/tobacco.

Table of Contents

Executive Summary v

1 Introduction 1

2 Methodology 3

3 Comprehensive Tobacco Control Programs 5

4 Target Audiences: Youth Only or General Population? 7
   Targeting adults and youth 7
   Targeting youth only. 7

5 Emotional Appeal 11
   Research findings on the importance of emotional appeal 11
   Research findings on emotional appeal of ads in media campaigns. 12

6 Message Content 15
   Health effects 16
   Tobacco industry deceptive practices 21
   Social approval/disapproval or refusal skills 26
   Secondhand smoke 28
   Cosmetic effects 29
   Addiction 30
   Athletic performance 30
   Individual choice 31
   Effectiveness of different message themes 32

7 Message Format 35
   Testimonials 35
   Graphic depiction. 36
   Celebrities. 36

8 Message Tone, Frequency, and Reach 39
   Humorous versus sad or serious tone 39
   Preachy tone. 40
   Ad frequency, reach, and duration. 40
   Integration of message elements. 42

9 Evaluation 43

Acknowledgments 45

References 47

Appendix 1: Case Histories of Campaigns with Effective Media Presence 51

Appendix 2: List of Advertisements by Country and U.S. State 53

Appendix 3: Research Summary 73

EXECUTIVE SUMMARY

Based on this review of material on youth tobacco use prevention campaigns from nine countries, the research literature, and extensive marketing program experience, we have drawn several conclusions about successful mass media campaigns.

In general, successful youth tobacco use prevention mass media campaigns:

- Are most effective when they are part of broader, comprehensive tobacco control programs designed to change a community's prevailing attitudes concerning tobacco use.

- Include ads with strong negative emotional appeal that produce, for example, a sense of loss, disgust, or fear.

- Introduce persuasive new information or new perspectives about health risks to smokers and nonsmokers.

- Use personal-testimony or graphic-depiction formats that youth find emotionally engaging but not authoritarian.

- Feature multiple message strategies, advertising executions, and media channels to consistently attract, engage, and influence diverse youth with varying levels of susceptibility to smoking.

- Provide adequate exposure to media messages over significant periods of time.

- Incorporate comprehensive formative, process, and outcome evaluation plans.

Specific conclusions and recommendations from each section of the report are provided below.

Comprehensive Programs

Mass media advertising to prevent youth tobacco use is most successful when it is part of a broader, comprehensive tobacco control initiative that includes such elements as taxes on tobacco products, curriculum-based school programs, cessation services, and grass-roots activism.

Mass media ads contribute to the synergy produced by different campaign elements working together to change a community's prevailing attitudes toward tobacco use.

Targeting Youth Versus the General Population

No clear consensus exists on whether ad campaigns that target youth audiences only or those directed at both adults and youth are more effective; both have been successful in changing youth attitudes and behaviors.

Some evidence indicates that older teens and youth who are most susceptible to smoking initiation may need specific, targeted tobacco counter-marketing messages. Those planning youth-targeted campaigns should consider developing messages that appeal to a broad range of youth, including high-risk youth and older teens who are more difficult to reach. Although evidence suggests that age-targeted messages can improve effectiveness, messages have been successfully developed to appeal to all ages, including adults.

Emotional Appeal

- Ads with strong and credible negative emotional appeal—leading the viewer to feel a sense of personal loss, sadness, anger, disgust, or fear—increase the attention to, and recall of, ads among youth audiences and enhance the ads' effectiveness.

- Emotionally compelling ads (such as personal testimonies) and those with strong graphic depictions run the risk of emotionally exhausting certain audience members if these ads are broadcast for significant periods of time. This has the potential to produce a defensive response to the message. Media schedules need to be designed to avoid emotional burnout.

Message Content

- *Health effects:* Ads that portray the serious health consequences of tobacco use in a credible manner can be effective. Health-effects information must be presented in innovative ways that engage viewers emotionally.

- *Tobacco industry deceptive practices:* Ads that communicate information on tobacco industry deceptive practices can be effective, but audiences probably need to be exposed over time to several different messages regarding tobacco industry behavior. To effectively communicate this message, the ads must educate the audience about tobacco industry marketing practices that attract youth to an addictive habit and do not reveal the serious negative consequences of smoking. These ads may be misunderstood by some youth, who question why a tobacco company should be treated differently from any other company because of its marketing practices. Only broadcast media campaigns conducted in the United States that use tobacco industry deceptive-practices ads have outcome evaluation results to date.

- *Social approval/disapproval or refusal skills:* Ads stressing that not smoking is socially acceptable or that smoking is negatively perceived by peers, and ads that introduce refusal skills, can be effective in increasing awareness of tobacco-related issues and reducing intention to smoke. However, the research indicating that these types of messages can be successful is limited primarily to controlled community trials. Results from one large-scale tobacco control program did not show success in changing behavior or attitudes toward smoking despite high awareness of campaign messages.

- *Secondhand smoke:* Secondhand-smoke ads inform youth about the potential for personal harm from exposure to the tobacco smoke of others. Limited data indicate that these ads can be effective among youth, but they have rarely been used as the only or major type of ad in a youth campaign. As a result, the influence of these types of ads has rarely been measured among youth.

- *Cosmetic effects, addiction, athletic performance:* Research on ads focusing on the short-term cosmetic effects of smoking, the addictive nature of tobacco, and the effects of smoking on athletic performance is limited. Available data suggest that ads emphasizing these themes are less effective among youth than ads that address the health effects of tobacco use or the deceptive practices of the tobacco industry.

- *Individual choice:* Individual-choice messages, which emphasize that youth have the choice of whether to smoke, have not been shown to be effective. Available data indicate that emphasizing the choice of whether to smoke without offering persuasive reasons not to smoke is not an effective strategy for preventing youth from using tobacco.

Message Format

- The testimonial, the personal story of someone who has experienced negative tobacco-related health or emotional consequences, is an effective message format. The testimonial format tends to elicit a strong emotional response in youth audiences, provides credible information about the negative effects of smoking, and has the added benefit of not telling the viewer what to do.

- Graphic depictions of the health effects of smoking are effective with youth audiences because these images can induce a strong emotional reaction (e.g., disgust or fear). But to be perceived as credible, the ads must depict the actual effects of smoking graphically and must present youth with information on the risks of smoking that they may not have considered before.

- The celebrity format should be used with caution. Although ads using celebrities are usually successful in attracting attention, they can create credibility concerns or other complications. Moreover, subsequent revelations of celebrity misdeeds can damage the impact of ad campaigns. The most effective celebrity ads seem to be those based on personal testimonials concerning the negative impact of tobacco use on the lives of celebrities or members of their families.

Message Tone, Frequency, and Reach

Youth respond more strongly to messages that produce negative emotions—feelings of loss, anger, sadness, fear, or disgust—than to humorous messages. Ads with a "preachy" tone that tell youth what to think and how to behave should be avoided. When ads offer advice and direction to youth, they may lead the audience to rebel against the message and produce the opposite of the desired result.

Messages will only be effective if audiences are adequately exposed to them. The messages must appear often enough for audiences to notice them, internalize them, and develop relevant attitude and behavior changes. Campaigns must maintain a strong and consistent presence in broadcast media to achieve program goals.

It is difficult, if not impossible, to disentangle the unique contribution of each message element (content, format, tone) to ad effectiveness. Careful attention to all message elements and ad execution (how the ad is created and presents the message) is essential; these elements must be integrated effectively to produce the desired impact.

Evaluation

Different aspects of youth tobacco use prevention mass media campaigns should be evaluated for these campaigns to succeed over time. Formative, process, and outcome evaluation activities need to be integrated into campaigns at each stage of ad development and implementation so that managers can develop the optimal communication strategies and respond to changes in target audience response over time.

INTRODUCTION

Globally, 4.9 million deaths a year are attributed to tobacco-related diseases (World Health Organization, 2005). If tobacco use continues unchecked, this rate is projected to rise to 10 million deaths annually by 2020. To help stem this alarming increase in tobacco-related mortality, governments should help reduce the number of young smokers because most smokers initiate tobacco use in their youth. One way to reduce the number of young smokers is to help youth make a commitment to not smoking (U.S. Department of Health and Human Services, 1994).

Mass media provide effective tools for convincing youth not to smoke, because they can communicate prevention messages directly to young people and influence their knowledge, attitudes, and behaviors (Hopkins et al., 2001). By using mass media as part of a comprehensive tobacco control program, several countries have been successful in reaching and influencing youth with messages that encourage a commitment to not smoking.

As part of its overall goal of reducing tobacco use, the Office on Smoking and Health of the Centers for Disease Control and Prevention (CDC) has prepared this report to build awareness of what the tobacco control community has learned about effective youth tobacco use prevention media campaigns. By combining field-based information with published research results, we aim to provide a collection of practical findings in a resource for those charged with developing and implementing effective mass media campaigns to reduce youth tobacco use.

Approach

We reviewed evaluation data on campaigns from Australia, Canada, England, Finland, the Netherlands, Norway, Poland, Scotland, and the United States. We summarize the elements of paid media campaigns in these countries that, based on available information from both published and unpublished sources, appear to have been most effective in changing youth attitudes about smoking, encouraging youth to commit to not smoking and, in some cases, reducing tobacco use. We focus on lessons learned about ad message content, format, and tone, as well as how often and how long ads should be aired. We also discuss the role of evaluation in developing effective media campaigns.

This is not a meta-analysis or a comprehensive review of the scientific literature on media campaigns in tobacco control. Rather, it is a review of selected studies and campaign information provided by researchers and practitioners in tobacco control programs who responded to a request for information or were identified through our efforts to find others involved in youth tobacco use prevention media campaigns in various countries.

We recognize that mass media are only part of the total plan needed to reduce youth tobacco use. School-based education and youth empowerment programs, and cessation programs, for example, can play important roles in the overall effectiveness of youth tobacco use prevention programs. However, evaluations of paid mass media campaigns, especially those focused on television ads, have produced the most consistent data available regarding message effectiveness. Therefore, in this review, we focus on findings from evaluations of television ads used in paid mass media campaigns.

We do not review other elements or types of comprehensive tobacco counter-marketing campaigns here. However, excellent reviews of the literature on tobacco use prevention and cessation and on overall tobacco control campaign effectiveness in the United States are available elsewhere (National Cancer Institute, 2000; CDC, 2000; Hopkins et al., 2001).

We also recognize that data on youth tobacco use prevention campaigns are too disparate and limited for drawing firm conclusions. We therefore highlight message strategies that, based on available data, generally appear to be most effective.

As states, national organizations, and countries develop their media campaigns, they need to choose the campaign elements that they expect will work most effectively with their target audiences and in their unique environments. These decisions should be based on their own message research and media campaign evaluations, as well as findings and recommendations from this and other reviews, such as those of Farrelly and colleagues (2003) and Wakefield and associates (2003).

This report has several limitations. First, cultural and ethnic differences are not explored; we draw conclusions only about the audiences targeted by the campaigns that we assessed. Second, additional evaluation data that we were unable to identify probably exist on youth tobacco use prevention campaigns in these and other countries, particularly developing countries.

Third, we focused on summarizing practical recommendations for program managers as well as research findings from published literature; we did not attempt a comprehensive review of the scientific literature on youth tobacco use prevention campaigns. Fourth, although we attempted to identify materials from youth tobacco use prevention media campaigns for all types of tobacco, the vast majority of the information we obtained pertained to cigarette smoking only. As a result, we do not specifically address prevention of the use of other forms of tobacco, such as smokeless tobacco or cigars.

A list of the campaigns and ads, including descriptions of the ad content and key messages, and a summary chart of the studies discussed in this report, are included as appendices to this document. For further information regarding the ads, please contact the CDC Office on Smoking and Health Media Campaign Resource Center at 770-488-5705, or send an e-mail to mcrc@cdc.gov.

Request

If you have conducted a youth tobacco use prevention media campaign and are willing to share lessons learned, please contact the Chief of the Health Communications Branch, Office on Smoking and Health, Mail Stop K-50, Centers for Disease Control and Prevention, 4770 Buford Highway NE, Atlanta, GA, USA 30341-3724.

METHODOLOGY

In June 2001, CDC and the World Health Organization (WHO) sent an international request through the Globalink listserv, whose members included approximately 2,000 tobacco control advocates from 80 countries, for information on youth tobacco use prevention mass media campaigns with documented results among youth. As part of this request, CDC and WHO asked for published and unpublished data from campaigns, such as consumer insight research; awareness, recall, and attitude evaluations; and data on smoking prevalence and cigarette consumption.

On behalf of CDC and WHO, we contacted people recognized by the tobacco control community as being involved in developing, implementing, or evaluating youth tobacco use prevention programs in one or more countries. A list of people who provided information for this report is included in the Acknowledgments, p. 45.

From June 2001 to August 2002, we collected campaign evaluation information from tobacco control organizations and researchers in Australia, Canada, England, Finland, Germany, the Netherlands, Norway, Poland, and the United States. Information on U.S. campaigns was contributed by the American Legacy Foundation and state organizations from Arizona, California, Florida, Massachusetts, Minnesota, Mississippi, Montana, New York, Oregon, Texas, Utah, and Vermont.

We included unpublished, so-called "gray" literature in this review because many useful tobacco control campaign evaluations are not published in the scientific literature and have much to offer.

Information on each of the mass media campaign evaluations reviewed in this report is available in Appendix 3.

We reviewed all of the information collected to identify the tobacco counter-advertising media campaign elements most commonly deemed effective in reaching and influencing youth audiences.

We based our conclusions on a synthesis of four types of information sources:

- Message research—studies in which participants rated the perceived effectiveness of ad content themes or actual ads (e.g., focus groups or classroom settings).

- Media campaign evaluations—quantitative, population-based studies of people exposed to ads aired in broad-scale tobacco counter-advertising campaigns targeted to specific geographic regions (states, provinces, countries) or broadcast in controlled community-based trials.

- Expert opinion—information gathered through interviews with people closely involved with ad campaigns and our own extensive public health, commercial marketing, and advertising experience.

- Selected aspects of the research literature that are relevant to the practical aspects of mass media anti-tobacco public health ad campaigns.

Each of the conclusions in this report is based on results from more than one geographic area. Data are limited in many cases, highlighting the need for more tobacco control programs to thoroughly evaluate their campaigns. Statistical significance of data (e.g., p values, 95% confidence intervals) was available from some sources and not others; such information is included when available. The methods and rigor of the campaign evaluations and the data and information sources used varied widely, preventing a formal empirical comparison of findings, such as a meta-analysis. As a result, the recommendations should be regarded as the perspectives of the authors, based on a careful review of available information from experienced campaign managers. The conclusions are intended to provide those responsible for developing media campaigns with practical suggestions for conducting effective youth tobacco use prevention advertising campaigns.

We judged message strategies to be most effective if their evaluations had several of the following characteristics:

- Results showing statistically significant differences in perceived effectiveness, awareness, beliefs and attitudes, and behavioral intent or reported behavior among youth using random sampling methodologies.

- Indications of an association between campaign ads and reduced smoking prevalence among youth.

- Similar results achieved in more than one geographic area.

- Direct comparisons showing that one message strategy was more effective than another.

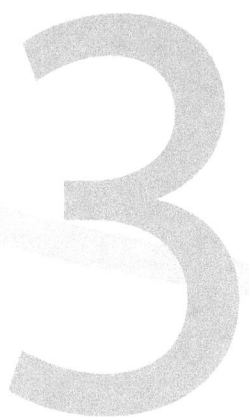

COMPREHENSIVE TOBACCO CONTROL PROGRAMS

Nearly all mass media campaigns that have achieved long-term success were implemented as part of a comprehensive tobacco control program. Campaigns in Finland, California, and Massachusetts were able to reduce smoking prevalence among adults and youth over time through this comprehensive approach (Biener et al., 2000; California Department of Health Services, 2000; Massachusetts Department of Public Health, 2000; Puska, 1999).

Several U.S. government and WHO reports note that mass media have played an important role in effective tobacco control programs when they were supported by other components of these programs, such as a mix of environmental and policy changes, educational programs, cessation treatment programs, and grassroots activism (U.S. Department of Health and Human Services, 2000; CDC, 1999; Hopkins et al., 2001; Institute of Medicine, 2000; WHO, 2001). When diverse tobacco control program elements work together to change the overall environment, they create a synergy that contributes to the success of mass media tobacco use prevention campaigns.

Specifically, mass media campaigns are most successful when they target people who are surrounded by anti-tobacco messages from several sources. For example, a mass media campaign is more likely to be effective with someone who frequents bars or restaurants that no longer allow smoking because of a community-wide clean air policy, is aware that the price of cigarettes has risen because of a tax increase, and has been told by a doctor about the dangers of tobacco use during a regular checkup, than with someone who has had none of these additional influences. The combined impact of these interventions is likely to cause a teen to think about the impact of tobacco use in his life and to make different decisions about tobacco use than if he had received only one of these messages.

We found that comprehensive tobacco control programs are necessary for success in youth-focused mass media campaigns as well. In several U.S. states, youth tobacco control programs were mandated by the legislatures or Master Settlement Agreement restrictions based on U.S. lawsuits against the tobacco industry. These states include Florida (Bauer et al., 2000; Bauer and Johnson, 2001), Minnesota (Minnesota Department of Health, 2002), Mississippi (Partnership for a Healthy Mississippi, 2001), and Texas (Texas Tobacco Prevention Initiative, 2001).

These youth-targeted tobacco use prevention campaigns were able to influence youth, effectively reducing uptake through strong media campaigns supported by community- and school-based programs, youth access policy enforcement and, in some cases, smoking cessation promotion. The media campaigns built awareness and delivered the message that youth needed to seriously consider not smoking, while the other tobacco control program elements provided additional incentives not to smoke, such as excise taxes that increased the cost of smoking, clean indoor air policies in schools and restaurants, and regulations that prohibited the sale of tobacco products to youth.

Conclusions

Research from several countries has consistently shown that tobacco counter-marketing campaigns are most successful when they are part of broader, comprehensive tobacco control activities in communities. These efforts may include such elements as environmental and policy changes, taxation, curriculum programs, cessation treatment programs, and grassroots activism. A key contributor to successful mass media campaigns is the synergy resulting from the different program elements working together to change society's prevailing attitudes about tobacco use.

4 TARGET AUDIENCES: YOUTH ONLY OR GENERAL POPULATION?

A frequent debate in the tobacco control field centers on the choice of whom to target with tobacco counter-marketing programs. Experts agree on the need to decrease smoking among youth (National Blueprint for Action, 2000), but not on the effectiveness of counter-marketing programs and messages directed toward youth compared with those that target the general population, including adults and youth.

Tobacco use usually begins in adolescence. For example, in the United States, about 70% of adult smokers report that they started smoking by the time they were 18 (CDC, 1994). Based on data from 131 countries, the Global Youth Tobacco Survey reports that 9% of 13- to 15-year-old students around the world currently smoke cigarettes (Warren et al., 2006).

Because most smokers begin using tobacco in adolescence, many program managers believe that tobacco use prevention campaigns should target youth. But other experts believe that targeting youth with prevention messages without communicating messages to the whole population drains resources from the real fight, which should focus on reducing and de-normalizing tobacco use among both adults and youth. These experts also believe that youth-oriented campaigns in isolation communicate a "forbidden fruit" message to youth, increasing their desire to engage in an activity that is prohibited for them but is acceptable for adults (Ling and Glantz, 2002; Atkin, 2000).

Targeting Adults and Youth

Campaigns in Australia, England, U.S./California, and U.S./Massachusetts were able to influence youth through comprehensive tobacco counter-marketing efforts targeting youth and adults (Biener et al., 2000; BMRB Social Research, 2002; California Department of Health Services, 2000; Hassard, 2000; Massachusetts Department of Public Health, 2000). Even though messages were not targeted specifically to them, youth reported equal or higher awareness of the campaigns compared with adults. They also reported learning new information, identifying with the ad messages, changing key attitudes and, in some cases, changing their smoking behaviors.

Targeting Youth Only

Tobacco control programs in U.S./Florida, U.S./Minnesota, and U.S./Mississippi, as well as the national program of the American Legacy Foundation, were able to change youth attitudes and behaviors associated with tobacco use by pursuing a strategy that targeted youth exclusively.

One of the challenges in developing effective anti-tobacco messages is achieving awareness and behavior change in youth who are most susceptible to smoking initiation (based on the number of friends and family members who smoke and the youths' attitudes toward tobacco and tobacco companies), including older youth. Several programs, including those of U.S./Arizona (Burgoon et al., 2000) and U.S./Florida (Sly, 1998), have found that older youth and those at higher risk of smoking initiation showed the least awareness of, and receptivity to, their messages. However, the American Legacy Foundation has been successful in creating messages that appealed equally to all youth (Farrelly MC, et al., 2002); responses to the messages from susceptible and older youth were similar to responses from younger and less susceptible youth. In Florida, the Legacy truth^{sm} ads evaluated in the same study were more influential across all youth, susceptible and non-susceptible, than any of the tobacco industry-sponsored youth prevention ads (RTI International, 2002). (For descriptions of the ads used in the campaigns described in this report, see Appendix 2.)

Those seeking to reach youth are well aware of the challenges of developing messages that communicate effectively to young people. Youth often discount messages that appear to speak to younger age groups, preferring to align themselves with an older age group that they perceive as being in a more desirable stage of life (Zollo, 1999). Young people are typically more responsive to ads that show people who are perceived as attractive and "cool" and are several years older than themselves. Programs such as the Target Market campaign in U.S./Minnesota have found that using teen members of the Target Market network (youth who voluntarily joined the state's counter-marketing initiative) as spokespeople in television ads was not successful (Ergo International, 2001). Other teens were not interested in watching or listening to youth who looked to be their own age or younger.

Targeting youth in general may not be enough to ensure campaign success among youth; campaigns may need to target specific segments of the youth population. For example, although Florida's program resulted in declines in smoking uptake and increased commitment to never smoking among middle school *and* high school audiences, the middle school students were the most responsive to certain program elements (Sly, 1998). The Minnesota Target Market campaign evaluation showed that campaign effectiveness among middle school students was much greater than among high school students (Ergo International, 2001). As a result, different strategies or messages from those used for middle school students may be needed to produce more significant changes in tobacco-related attitudes among high school students.

U.S./Mississippi decided to develop ads targeted to youth of different ages instead of trying to develop ads that would appeal to all youth (Partnership for a Healthy Mississippi, 2001). These ads capitalized on attitude differences between age groups that were identified through qualitative research. The ages of 6–11 years were defined as the "age of reason," when youth willingly accept information about the risks of tobacco use and directions to speak with those they love about quitting. The ages of 12–17 years were defined as the "age of rebellion," when youth resist advice from authority figures but accept factual information to consider when making their own independent decisions. The Partnership developed "age of reason" ads that gave younger viewers advice and direction on how to avoid the effects of tobacco-related diseases on their lives. "Age of rebellion" ads gave older youth facts about smoking and tobacco industry behavior that would encourage them to question the value of using tobacco. Mississippi youth behavior risk surveys found that smoking in both age groups declined, indicating that targeting by age could be an effective strategy (Partnership for a Healthy Mississippi, 2000).

However, some programs have been successful in developing messages that appeal to youth of different ages. The advertising messages of the American Legacy truth[sm] campaign resonated well with youth aged 12–17 years as well as with young adults aged 18–24 years (Farrelly MC, et al., 2002). Aided awareness, participants' ability to remember an ad when it is described to them, was slightly higher among youth than young adults, but levels among both populations were high. However, receptivity, or message appeal and acceptance, declined among both audiences (although it declined slightly more among young adults) as the message focused less on tobacco industry deceptive practices and long-term health risks and more on short-term health effects and individual choice.

Conclusions

No clear consensus exists on whether to target youth only or the general population with tobacco use prevention campaigns. Some research indicates that youth-targeted tobacco control programs in general, and youth-targeted mass media campaigns specifically, can be successful in developing awareness and changing attitudes and behaviors associated with tobacco use. However, other research indicates that campaigns targeted to the general population can also reduce smoking among youth.

Some evidence indicates that older teens and youth who are most susceptible to smoking initiation are less responsive to typical tobacco counter-advertising messages than other youth (Hassard, 2000; Sly et al., 2001). Messages need to appeal to youth of all ages, including subgroups that are harder to reach. Tobacco counter-advertising messages should either target different age groups separately or use themes that resonate broadly with youth of different ages.

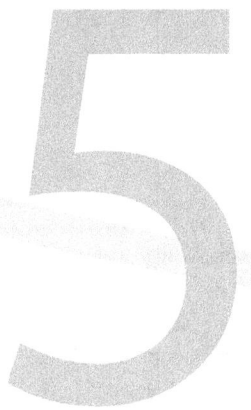

EMOTIONAL APPEAL

Decades of research in communication, behavioral science, advertising, and marketing have shown that the most effective ads generate some level of emotional response among audiences. According to the Elaboration Likelihood Model of persuasion (Petty and Cacioppo, 1986), ads must first gain the attention of the audience, most of whom have a low level of involvement or interest in the topic (in this case, tobacco use prevention or cessation) before the communication process can begin. Emotional messages are better remembered than non-emotional ones (Lang, 1995), and emotional appeals, which engage the viewer on a personal level, tend to be more effective in gaining audience attention than strictly cognitive appeals that rely on a rational, directive approach (e.g., providing tobacco health facts or encouraging viewers to "just say no" to smoking) (Petty and Cacioppo, 1986).

Evidence increasingly shows that engaging viewers emotionally in the tobacco use prevention message is important to an ad's overall effectiveness (Biener et al., 2002). The need to engage viewers emotionally has been an accepted tenet of consumer advertising for some time, but research demonstrating its applicability to tobacco control has lagged behind research focusing on message content (Biener et al., 2004).

Although the emotional approach traditionally used in tobacco control and other public health ad campaigns has been based on fear, it is the ability to arouse any one of a number of negative emotional responses—such as anger, sadness, disgust, loss, or fear—that increases a message's effectiveness (Biener et al., 2002). Negative emotions that an effective tobacco prevention ad may arouse include fear of the health consequences of smoking, a sense of personal loss or sadness due to the death or illness of a loved one, or anger at tobacco companies because of their deceptive marketing practices (Biener et al., 2002).

Research Findings on the Importance of Emotional Appeal

Several studies have examined the role and effectiveness of generating an emotional response in youth tobacco counter-marketing messages. In the Teen Research Unlimited (TRU) multistate focus group study, for example, youth rated a series of tobacco use prevention ads according to whether the ads would make them "stop and think about not using tobacco" (Teen Research Unlimited, 1999). Three of the four ads rated by youth as most likely to make them consider not using tobacco generated strong negative emotional responses focused on a sense of loss or fear associated with smoking-related illnesses.

The highest rated ads were those that highlighted the health consequences of tobacco use, typically in a dramatic or emotional way, by portraying smokers with tobacco use-related diseases describing their fear of not being able to breathe, or the grief of losing a loved one to a tobacco-related disease. The ads with the lowest ratings were tobacco industry-sponsored tobacco use prevention ads, such as the Philip Morris Company's Think. Don't Smoke. ads, which have been characterized by researchers as having low emotional engagement because they do not challenge or engage the viewer's beliefs or feelings (Teen Research Unlimited, 1999; Wakefield, 2002). These Philip Morris ads, which have a personal-choice theme, present smoking as a rational choice young people can make, but they do not include information about the serious negative consequences of tobacco use.

In the Youth Appraisal of Anti-smoking Advertising study, 278 8th-, 10th-, and 12th-grade students in Boston and Chicago appraised a broad range of 50 anti-smoking ads produced in the United States from 1997 to 2001. The students rated the ads produced by the tobacco companies as less engaging, less confrontational, and having less negative emotional content than ads produced by state and national tobacco control programs. As a result, youth would be less likely to think about the message content of these ads in a personal way that would affect their attitudes or behavior regarding tobacco use (Wakefield et al., 2002).

The participants in this study were also asked 1 week after seeing the ads to identify the ads that they recalled best, had discussed with others outside of the rating session, and had thought most about. Ads that included personal testimonials or that had a negative visceral element (inducing an "ugh" response) were significantly more likely to be recalled, discussed, and identified as making youth "stop and think" at follow-up (Wakefield, 2003).

In an extension of this study to Australia and Great Britain using the same protocol, youth in these countries rated the ads similarly to youth in the United States (Wakefield et al., 2003). Consistent with the Elaboration Likelihood Model (Petty and Caccioppo, 1986), ads that included moving personal testimonials and graphic negative elements were consistently more likely to be recalled and discussed, and to make youth "stop and think" than ads presenting personal-choice messages (the type of ad typically developed by the tobacco industry).

Tobacco company-sponsored tobacco use prevention ads, such as the Philip Morris Think. Don't Smoke. ads (see Appendix 2 for descriptions of these and other ads discussed in this report), have not been found effective in changing youth beliefs, attitudes, and behavior associated with tobacco use (see individual-choice discussion, page 31). The Youth Appraisal of Anti-smoking Advertising research suggests that the low impact of industry-sponsored tobacco use prevention ads is probably due to a lack of characteristics that engage youth emotionally and promote processing of information contained in the ad (Wakefield, 2002; Wakefield et al., 2003).

Research Findings on Emotional Appeal of Ads in Media Campaigns

Several researchers have assessed the effectiveness of anti-smoking ads designed to evoke an emotional response in adolescents in actual campaigns. These studies have found that campaigns using ads with strong emotional appeals are effective in influencing tobacco-related beliefs, attitudes, and behaviors among youth.

The Norway Youth Provocative Appeals campaign evaluation was a longitudinal study from 1992 to 1995 that targeted adolescents aged 14–15 years living in southeastern Norway. Researchers developed provocative anti-smoking messages designed to prevent the onset of smoking among adolescents. They communicated these messages through mass media and evaluated the effectiveness of these messages in preventing smoking and encouraging cessation among adolescents (Hafstad et al., 1997). The researchers based their work on a mass communication theory that supports the use of emotional appeals when awareness of a problem is high, interest is low, and no new information is available to offer on the subject (Rothschild, 1987).

Although some public health communication experts discourage messages that could be perceived as "blaming the victim," the Norwegian researchers began their media campaign with a message that, "Girls are stupid because the more we know about the health risks of smoking, the more Norwegian girls start to smoke." They decided to target girls because, although smoking prevalence was decreasing overall in Norway, it was higher among adolescent girls and young women than among boys and young men. In its second year, the campaign focused on young females with a message that smoking was due to poor self-control and endangered the environment. The message in the third year targeted young men and women, suggesting that smokers had less successful lives than nonsmokers (Hafstad et al., 1997).

The researchers found that among nonsmokers, a significantly lower percentage of boys and girls exposed to the mass media campaign started to smoke (8.6%) than in the control area (12.4%). Also, significantly more girls exposed to the campaign who had been smokers at the beginning of the study had stopped smoking (25.6%) than girls in the control area (17.6%). The Norwegian researchers concluded that provocative messages that emotionally engage adolescents were effective in preventing the onset of smoking among young females in southeastern Norway, but cautioned that this approach could be rejected by the target audience in other cultures (Hafstad et al., 1997).

In the U.S./Massachusetts tobacco surveys, 8 ads were chosen for study from approximately 100 ads used in the state mass media campaign (Biener et al., 2004). The ads used a broad spectrum of messages, including normative behavior or social acceptance, illness related to tobacco use, and the deceptive practices of the tobacco industry. The ads also ranged in emotional tone from humorous to serious. An independent panel of youth had previously sorted the ads into groups according to message type and emotional tone (Table 1). A second group of youth evaluated the ads according to the extent to which they could recall the ad after hearing a description of it, as well as the ad's perceived effectiveness (Table 2).

In the follow-up surveys, youth were more likely to recall and perceive as effective anti-smoking ads that generated negative emotions (fear, sadness) than ads that generated positive emotions (happiness, humor, amusement) (Table 2). The four ads rated as most effective scored highest on the negative-emotion scale (sad and frightening) and highest on cognitive quality (interesting, thought-provoking, and believable). All of these ads depicted illness and suffering resulting from smoking, and three of the four ads criticized the tobacco industry's practices.

Table 1

Characteristics of Eight Anti-Tobacco Ads Broadcast in U.S./Massachusetts, 1993–1998

Ads	Negative Emotion*	Positive Emotion*	Strength of Emotional Appeal*	Cognitive Quality*
Happy Birthday	4.9	2.4	5.0	5.2
Pam Laffin	4.9	1.8	5.3	5.4
Janet Sackman	4.7	1.7	5.0	5.3
Cowboy	4.6	1.8	4.9	5.1
Camel	1.4	4.5	2.6	3.2
Lung/Dinner	2.7	4.7	3.4	3.5
Monica	2.0	2.6	3.1	3.9
Models	1.4	2.7	2.9	3.8

* Mean scale values as rated by panel of 104 youth judges (1 = low, 7 = high)

Note: Differences in strength of emotional appeal and cognitive quality scores were statistically significant for each of the illness ads compared with all the humorous and normative or social acceptance ads based on non-overlapping 95% confidence intervals. (Biener et al., 2004)

Table 2

Recall and Perceived Effectiveness of Anti-Tobacco Ads Broadcast in U.S./Massachusetts, 1993–1998, by Message Type

Message Type	Overall Recall (%)*	Perceived Effectiveness†
Illness Ads	68.4	8.2
Humorous Ads	69.3	6.8
Normative or Social Acceptance Ads	42.2	6.4

* Survey respondents who recalled seeing an ad when given a brief description of it.
† Based on recall, where 0 = not a good ad and 10 = a good ad.

Note: Differences were statistically significant at $p < 0.05$, when overall results for illness ads were compared with those of normative or social acceptance ads, and when overall recall for the humorous ads was compared with that of normative or social acceptance ads. Scores for perceived effectiveness were statistically significant at $p < 0.05$ for the illness ads compared with both humorous and normative or social acceptance ads. (Biener et al., 2004)

Although emotional appeal can be a very important component of effective anti-tobacco ads for youth, invoking too much emotion can limit the length of time for which an ad can be used. An internal agency memo from Arnold Communications, Boston, cited by the U.S./Massachusetts tobacco control program staff, indicated that the testimonial *Pam Laffin* and *Rick Stoddard* ads achieved saturation (the point at which the viewing audience no longer paid attention to the ads or received any additional benefit from their messages) after being broadcast for only 7–11 weeks (Brogdon, oral communication, 2000). Viewers contacted the tobacco control program to request that the ads be discontinued because of their intense emotional content. Those who complained about the *Pam Laffin* and *Rick Stoddard* ads said that they could not bear to watch them anymore; they had quickly understood the strong message and did not need or want to see the ads again and again. These highly emotional ads were found to build high levels of awareness among audiences much more quickly than other ads (Brogdon, oral communication, 2000). Subsequent media schedules shortened the number of weeks for which these ads were broadcast to avoid emotionally exhausting audiences and reducing ad effectiveness.

Similarly, researchers in Poland used the Every Cigarette Is Doing You Damage campaign to provide mass media support for the Great Polish Smokeout program in 1999. Television stations reported that viewers called to complain that they were distressed by the graphic nature of the ads, especially when the ads were aired during the dinner hour. After the tobacco control programs shared data with the television stations indicating that these ads were effective in influencing youth audiences, the television station managers allowed the ads to stay on the air (Przewozniak et al., 2002).

Conclusions

Generating a strong negative emotional response can be an effective component of youth tobacco use prevention ads. The research reviewed for this report confirms findings from a substantial body of literature showing that strong negative emotional appeals increase the attention to, and recall of, ads among youth audiences as well as overall effectiveness. But while emotionally compelling ads (especially those with personal testimonies about the negative impact of tobacco-related illness and death of loved ones) can be effective, they run the risk of emotionally exhausting certain audience members. Adjustments may need to be made to ad placement schedules, such as airing them for shorter periods of time, to avoid this problem.

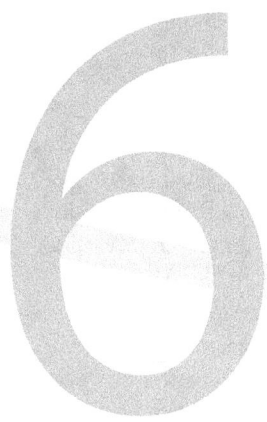

6 MESSAGE CONTENT

The research community has not reached consensus on how the messages most commonly communicated by tobacco use prevention ads should be categorized (Farrelly et al., 2003; Wakefield et al., 2003; Goldman and Glantz, 1998). We have chosen to categorize the message content of the ads reviewed using groupings most commonly employed by researchers, while recognizing that some ads may belong to more than one category. In this report, we discuss only content themes for which data on effectiveness in youth are available.

In the following sections, we review the results of evaluation research on ads whose messages focus on one of the following themes:

- *Health effects:* The most common content of youth tobacco use prevention ad messages is the adverse health effects of smoking. These ads typically attempt to communicate one or more of the health problems associated with smoking, often presenting information that viewers are unlikely to know or perspectives that viewers are unlikely to have considered previously. These ads typically portray the negative consequences of these health effects on smokers and their loved ones.

- *Tobacco industry deceptive practices:* Ads providing information on the deceptive practices of the tobacco industry, such as denying the health effects of tobacco use, were first introduced in California in 1990 as part of a tobacco de-normalization strategy intended to reduce the societal acceptance of tobacco use. These ads are designed to reduce the glamour associated with smoking and to make audiences aware of how the tobacco industry is misleading consumers into addiction. Such messages typically portray the industry as composed of uncaring, greedy, and manipulative corporations willing to sell hazardous and addictive products for financial gain.

- *Social approval or disapproval and refusal skills:* Some messages about social approval of not smoking or disapproval of smoking, as well as refusal-skills messages, emphasize that instead of increasing the popularity of youth, smoking has just the opposite effect. Other ads address ways to respond to peer pressure to smoke.

- *Secondhand smoke:* Secondhand-smoke messages stress the effects of cigarette smoke on nonsmokers or steps that can be taken to reduce exposure to secondhand smoke.

- *Adverse cosmetic effects:* Messages about adverse cosmetic effects emphasize the short-term effects of smoking on appearance, such as bad breath or discolored teeth. These ads typically stress the disapproval of peers that results from these effects of smoking on one's appearance.

- *Addiction:* Addiction messages stress the potential for youth to become addicted to tobacco use.

- *Athletic performance:* Athletic-performance messages address the adverse impact of smoking on a youth's performance in a sport.

- *Individual choice:* Individual-choice messages emphasize that youth can make independent decisions about whether to smoke.

Health Effects

Mass Media Campaign Evaluations

Australia

The Australia National Tobacco Campaign survey results demonstrated that young audiences were, in some cases, more receptive to graphic portrayals of newly understood health risks of smoking than adults. Although the Every Cigarette is Doing You Damage (ECIDYD) campaign targeted adults, follow-up surveys showed that, for some measures, the response of teenagers (aged 14–17 years) was greater than that of adults (Hassard, 2000).

- Awareness of the campaign was greater among teen-aged smokers and teenaged recent quitters (96%) than adult smokers and adult recent quitters (87%).

- Teenaged smokers and recent quitters who had viewed the campaign ads showed similar levels of agreement with the basic messages of the campaign to those of adult smokers and adult recent quitters.

Regarding the basic campaign message that, "Every cigarette is doing you damage":

- 97% of teenaged smokers and recent quitters agreed that the message represented the truth, compared with 81% of adult smokers and recent quitters.

- 82% of teenaged smokers and recent quitters believed the statement "smoking causes strokes" to be true, compared with 77% of adults.

- Teens and adults had similar belief ratings about smoking causing blood clots in the brain (73% and 71%, respectively) and decay in the lungs (94% and 94%, respectively).

- 85% of teenaged smokers and recent quitters believed that smoking blocks arteries with fatty deposits, compared with 76% of adults.

Note: Conclusions should be evaluated as directional because of the relatively small number of teenagers who were recent quitters.

Researchers compared youth responses to the national ECIDYD campaign with results from the Australia Health Omnibus Survey, which evaluated the Stressing Out campaign created for a youth audience by the South Australian Smoking and Health Project (Hassard, 2000). Although awareness of the two campaigns was similar, teenagers were more influenced by the ECIDYD campaign, which focused on health risks, than the Stressing Out campaign, which focused on short-term consequences of smoking. Almost 54% of the youth surveyed strongly agreed with the message presented in the ECIDYD campaign, but only 35% agreed with the short-term–consequences message in the Stressing Out campaign. About 61% of youth smokers surveyed reported that the ECIDYD ads made them more likely to quit, compared with only 31% of youth for the Stressing Out ads (Hassard, 2000).

Canada/British Columbia

Results from the Canadian Tobacco Use Monitoring Survey showed that the prevalence of current smoking in British Columbia among people aged 15 years or older dropped from 26% in 1997 to 20% in 1999 (Lavack, 2001). This decrease followed the conclusion of a 2-year, multi-level anti-smoking campaign in British Columbia that used a mix of messages in the broadcast media primarily focused on the health risks of smoking (British Columbia Ministry of Health, 2000). Several of the ads were produced by U.S. states and featured people who had suffered from the negative health effects of smoking; one ad discussed the number of British Columbians affected by tobacco-related illnesses. The media campaign was also supported by Critics' Choice, a school-based program that reached approximately two thirds of British Columbia students aged 10–17 years, and by the secondhand-smoke workers' compensation board regulation, enacted in 1998 to eliminate smoking in workplaces. The smoking prevalence for youth aged 15–19 years continued to drop, declining from 20% in 1999 to 18% in 2000 (British Columbia Ministry of Health, 2000).

Poland

Poland used the Australia-developed ECIDYD campaign for the mass media portion of the Great Polish Smokeout program in 1999. The post-campaign evaluation of adult and youth (aged 13–15 years) audiences showed that youth had higher awareness of the ads than adults, and higher levels of agreement about the ads' relevance and thought-provoking ability; their level of agreement about the ads' believability was almost as high (Table 3) (Przewozniak et al., 2002).

Table 3

Poland ECIDYD Campaign Youth and Adult Responses

Ad	Awareness (%)		Believability (%)		Relevance (%)		Thought Provoking (%)	
	Youth	Adult	Youth	Adult	Youth	Adult	Youth	Adult
Lung	66	43	88	96	70	62	75	62
Tumour	75	40	87	92	68	58	75	62
Artery	67	32	86	90	67	63	72	69
Brain	66	19	83	94	66	61	73	65

(Przewozniak et al., 2002)

England

England's Testimonials campaign encouraged smokers to quit by showing emotional pain of smokers and their families due to smoking-related illness and death. After viewing the ads *Stephen* and *Rebecca*, which featured two people who had suffered health consequences from smoking, more youth than adults reported learning about the health effects of smoking. Of youth surveyed in the England Anti-smoking Advertising Tracking Survey, 84% realized that not only old people suffer from smoking-related illnesses, compared with 75% of adults. Ninety percent of youth agreed that it is important to keep trying to quit smoking, compared with 76% of adults. Although the campaign targeted adults, 38% of youth stated that they could identify with the people and situations in the ads, compared with 70% of adults (BMRM Social Research, 2002).

U.S./Arizona

The University of Arizona conducted the Arizona Tobacco Education and Prevention Program (TEPP) media campaign evaluation to determine the effectiveness of an ad called *Doesn't Kill*. They also gathered data on participant awareness of, and reactions to, the American Legacy Foundation's truth[sm] campaign ads, which focused mainly on tobacco industry deceptive practices and were aired during the same period. In the *Doesn't Kill* ad, several teenagers announce that tobacco did not kill their parents or friends as everyone thought it would; the ad then shows that each parent or friend suffered major negative physical consequences from tobacco use. A description of the truth[sm] ads is available in Table 4 (University of Arizona, 2000).

Although the intent of the Arizona TEPP research was not to compare the efficacy of the two types of ads, comparisons are possible. Teens did not like the *Doesn't Kill* ad as well as most of the truth[sm] ads, but significantly more respondents agreed that the *Doesn't Kill* ad was more likely to make teenagers think about quitting smoking than any of the other ads or groups of ads (Table 5) (University of Arizona, 2000).

Table 4

truth[sm] U.S./National Campaign Ad Descriptions

Ad	Ad Description
truth 1	A series of ads portraying a teenager reading e-mail messages sent to the truth.com Web site that address some of youths' questions about truth[sm] and the tobacco issue.
truth 2	A series of ads portraying teenagers holding electric counters flashing numbers pertaining to important tobacco issues, such as tobacco industry spending on marketing and number of deaths from tobacco.
truth 3	A series of ads portraying teens trying a variety of experiences and products, such as bungee jumping, slam dunking a basketball, and driving rental cars. A narrator says that tobacco is the only product or experience that kills one out of three people who use it.
truth 4	An ad portraying teenagers driving around a wealthy neighborhood trying to hypnotize people who work for tobacco companies to make them feel better about their unethical work.
truth 5	An ad portraying teenagers piling hundreds of body bags outside a large building to illustrate the number of people who die every day from tobacco.

(University of Arizona, 2000)

Table 5

U.S./Arizona Youth Response to *Doesn't Kill* and truth[sm] Ads

Response	Ads Reviewed (% who agree or strongly agree)					
	Doesn't Kill	truth 1	truth 2	truth 3	truth 4	truth 5
I like this ad or series of ads.	79.8	88.3	85.6	85.8	85.0	92.7
The people who made this ad are smart.	93.4	90.6	93.5	90.6	83.3	94.5
This ad will make teenagers think about quitting smoking.	95.7	88.2	87.2	77.0	59.1	85.4
I like this ad more than most others I have seen.	69.7	72.4	73.7	74.7	57.6	70.3

(University of Arizona, 2000)

Table 6

Recognition and Impact Comparison of Anti-Smoking Ads by U.S./Utah Youth

TV Ad	% Recognition	% Influenced
Debi	72	43
Teenagers in local Utah settings talk about why they do not smoke	91	23
Pam Laffin	67	8
Cowboy	57	7
Teenagers at Great Salt Lake talk about why they started smoking	60	5
Janet Sackman	35	5

Note: Percentage influenced by *Debi* ad was significantly higher than for all other ads. (Nieger et al., 2002)

U.S./Massachusetts

The Massachusetts Department of Health's tobacco control program used a comprehensive tobacco de-normalization approach instead of a targeted youth campaign. University of Massachusetts Boston researchers used the Massachusetts tobacco surveys to evaluate the recall and persuasiveness of anti-smoking mass media messages aired by the Massachusetts Department of Health in 1999. Before the survey, small panels of teens categorized the ads based on message content (See Appendix 3 for specifics) (Biener, 2002).

Respondents to the survey rated the ads on a scale of 0 to 10, with 0 indicating that the ad was a poor anti-smoking ad and 10 indicating that it was a good anti-smoking ad. Mean ratings for ads depicting illness (8.3) and tobacco industry deceptive practices (8.1) were significantly higher than ratings for the ads focused on sports performance, social acceptance, and being cool (7.0). Ads aired by the Philip Morris Company that focused on individual choice received the lowest average rating (5.8) (Biener, 2002).

The Massachusetts researchers reported that youth smoking prevalence for high school students dropped from 36% in 1995 to 30% in 1999 (Abt Associates, 2000). The researchers concluded that, "Youth prevention programs should not shy away from tobacco counter-advertising ads that feature the serious [health] consequences of smoking." These types of ads are the ones perceived as most effective by teenagers, regardless of their smoking status, age, gender, or ethnicity (Biener, 2002).

U.S./Utah

In 1998, the Utah Department of Health used four television ads produced in other states as well as several new locally produced ads in its youth anti-tobacco media campaign. Results from the Utah Tobacco Media Campaign evaluation indicated that *VoiceBox/Debi* (a health effects ad) had the greatest influence on teens' decisions not to smoke, and had the second highest level of recall (Table 6). The most recognizable ad was one produced locally that depicted Utah teenagers and prominent young adults near familiar local landmarks. But this local message, which featured positive testimony about reasons not to smoke, had about half the impact of the *VoiceBox/Debi* ad in influencing youths' intent not to smoke (Neiger et al., 2002).

Message Research

Canada/British Columbia

A youth education program in Canada, Critics' Choice, offered students the chance to view a series of anti-smoking ads and vote for the ad that was most likely to prevent them from starting to smoke or to encourage smokers to quit (perceived effectiveness) (British Columbia Ministry of Health, 2000). In all 4 years of the program, students chose ads that graphically portrayed the health consequences of smoking as those most likely to influence youth to avoid smoking or consider quitting. In 1997, participants chose

VoiceBox/Debi as most likely to influence their smoking-related behaviors; in 1998, *Artery*; in 1999, *Stroke*; and in 2000, *Tar Lung* (British Columbia Department of Health, 2000).

U.S./National

In 1997, the CDC sponsored U.S./National quantitative copy testing that compared the *Cowboy* ad, which depicts the health effects of smoking, with *Models*, in which players on the women's U.S. Olympic soccer team communicate about the ability to perform better in sports if one does not smoke. The ad scores were also compared with the average scores of thousands of other ads previously tested by consumer products companies using the same methodology. Results indicated that ad recall, main message recall, and key measures, such as ability to convince or engage the viewer, were better for *Cowboy* than for *Models*, and that *Cowboy* scored above average on most key measures. When the verbatim comments were analyzed to determine the reasons for *Cowboy*'s popularity, the emotional story about the cowboy's death and the loss to his brother, as well as the graphic images of the cowboy's last days in a hospital bed, were the elements of the ad most often mentioned by respondents (Gutierrez, personal communication, 1998).

U.S./Multistate

In 1999, four state tobacco control programs joined CDC to evaluate 10 anti-smoking ads, including two produced by the tobacco industry, for their impact on youth audiences. The Teen Research Unlimited (TRU) multistate focus groups consisted of 20 at-risk youth focus groups conducted in Massachusetts, California, and Arizona. Participants indicated which of 10 ads would most make them "stop and think about not using tobacco."

Three of the ads with the highest ratings by the focus groups presented stories about the negative consequences of smoking on real people and all four of these ads graphically showed the consequences of smoking (loss of larynx, emphysema, hospitalization, seizures, death). The adolescents appeared to have been more strongly affected by the idea of living with the negative consequences of tobacco than by the idea of dying from them (Teenage Research Unlimited, 1999).

U.S./North Carolina

Researchers at the University of North Carolina conducted four focus groups in that state using the same methodology and the same set of ads as in the multistate research. The North Carolina Anti-smoking Ad Focus Groups findings in 2000 were virtually identical to those of the TRU study (University of North Carolina, 2002).

Another study by the University of North Carolina (2002) showed that teens were becoming increasingly aware and critical of tobacco counter-marketing messages. However, the messages that described the serious health consequences of tobacco use, including the impact of secondhand smoke, were perceived by teens as most likely to cause viewers to stop and think about the dangers of tobacco use (University of North Carolina, 2002).

U.S/California

The 1998 Protection Motivation Theory Message Study by University of California, Irvine researchers found that ads focusing on the serious health consequences of tobacco use could have the reverse of the intended effect in certain audiences. The researchers showed 2,800 7th- and 10th-grade students 194 anti-smoking television ads in use from 1986 to 1997 to evaluate the impact of the ads on intentions to smoke and on smoking-related beliefs (Pechmann et al., 2003). Messages about the serious health effects of smoking strengthened beliefs that smoking poses severe health risks, but failed to reduce intentions to smoke. When data from the teens who felt most invulnerable to health risks were examined separately, the researchers found that the stronger the teens' perceptions that smoking poses severe health risks, the stronger their intent to smoke, apparently due to the appeal of tobacco as "forbidden fruit" (Pechmann et al., 2003).

This study also found that health-risk and addiction ads can lessen the intention to smoke, but only if they stress the fact that youth are susceptible to the health risks of smoking. To emphasize health risk vulnerability, the researchers recommended that ads tell true-life stories of younger victims, stressing how quickly these victims became addicted to smoking, and show how much they have suffered from their illness or from the illnesses of those they love (Pechmann et al., 2003).

U.S./Utah

In 1998, the Utah Department of Health conducted formative message research using tobacco prevention ads developed in other tobacco control programs to evaluate which messages might be most effective among Utah youth. The results indicated that Utah youth aged 11–18 years were most interested in, and persuaded by, ads that used a real-life format, such as testimonials from people who had experienced tobacco-related health effects. In follow-up focus groups, the youth were not shocked or offended by the new information shared in the ads about how tobacco companies were targeting them. The youth also dismissed ads that depicted what they perceived as unlikely events. For example, they responded, "that would never happen," after viewing an ad showing cigarettes raining down out of the sky to communicate that tobacco companies are targeting youth (Murphy, 2000).

Tobacco Industry Deceptive Practices

Mass Media Campaign Evaluations

U.S./National—American Legacy Foundation

The American Legacy Foundation's truth^{sm} campaign is a national U.S. media effort that began in 1999 to prevent tobacco use among youth (aged 12–17 years), particularly those most susceptible to tobacco use. The campaign is based on research indicating that at-risk youth often begin to smoke because this behavior communicates a level of freedom, risk-taking, and defiance that they find attractive (U.S. Department of Health and Human Services, 1994). The Legacy ads show authority-defying youth from diverse ethnic and socioeconomic backgrounds uncovering facts about tobacco industry activities and actions. Many of these ads also address the adverse health consequences of tobacco use. Probably one of the best known Legacy ads is *Body Bags*, in which youth place 1,200 bags representing human bodies outside the headquarters of a tobacco company to demonstrate the daily death toll in the United States from smoking. While the Legacy ads were airing, the tobacco industry aired youth tobacco use prevention ads with an individual-choice theme.

Through the Legacy Media Tracking Surveys (LMTS), the Foundation evaluated the target audience response to the broadcast campaign. The Legacy ads were rated highly for receptivity (based on whether the ad was perceived as convincing, captured viewers' attention, or gave good reasons not to smoke, and on whether viewers talked to a friend about the ad) among smoking and nonsmoking youth, and across races and ethnicities, with nearly 90% of youth aged 12–17 years reporting that the ads were convincing and gave them good reasons not to smoke (Farrelly et al., 2002). Comparisons of the Legacy ads to individual-choice ads produced by the tobacco industry showed that the industry-sponsored ads were significantly less well received by youth who were current smokers or most susceptible to smoking (Table 7). Of the five message types tested, the ads combining messages about tobacco industry deceptive practices with health-risk information had the highest receptivity and unaided recall ratings (the ability to remember the ad without assistance) among youth and young adults.

The recall numbers identified through the LMTS are especially striking because respondents were more than six times more likely to remember the Legacy ads than tobacco industry-sponsored ads (Farrelly et al., 2002). Furthermore, nearly 75% of respondents in this study could remember seeing at least one Legacy ad compared with 66% for any of the tobacco industry ads, even though the tobacco industry spent considerably more money purchasing broadcast ad placements than the Legacy Foundation (Farrelly et al., 2002).

Analyses of the nationally representative U.S. Monitoring the Future (MTF) adolescent surveys showed significant declines in current smoking prevalence among students in grades 8, 10, and 12 from 1999 through 2002 that were associated with exposure to the truth^{sm} campaign (Farrelly et al., 2005). The relative decline in smoking prevalence was 3.2% annually from 1997 to 1999, increasing to 6.8% annually from 2000 to 2002. Overall, an estimated 22% of the decline in adolescent smoking was attributable to the truth^{sm} ad campaign. The findings from these analyses demonstrated a dose-response relationship, with those students with higher estimated levels of exposure to campaign ads experiencing a larger relative decline in smoking prevalence compared to those with lower estimated levels of ad exposure. The dose-response findings were more consistent among 8th grade students compared to those in 10th and 12th grades.

Table 7

Receptivity and Unaided Awareness for Legacy and Philip Morris U.S./National Youth Tobacco Use Prevention Ads

Ad	Description	Receptivity Rating by Respondents*	
		Youth (12–17)	Young Adults (18–24)
Legacy *Body Bags*	Industry deceptive practices with health risks	3.1	3.0
Legacy *Daily Dose*	Industry deceptive practices with health risks	3.0	2.8
Legacy *Beach*	Industry deceptive practices, humor	2.9	2.7
Philip Morris *Karate Kid*	Short-term health effects, shortness of breath, affecting physical performance	2.8	2.5
Philip Morris *Boy on the Bus*	Individual choice	2.4	2.2

*Ads were rated based on four factors, with one point given for each factor considered to be present: convincing, grabbed attention, gave good reasons not to smoke, talked to friends. Differences between the Individual Choice and Industry Deceptive Practices ads were statistically significant at 95% confidence intervals. (Farrelly et al., 2002)

Note: 47% of respondents were able to recall the Legacy *Body Bags*, *Daily Dose*, and *Beach* ads without assistance, compared with 6.5% for the Philip Morris Think. Don't Smoke. *Karate Kid* and *Boy on the Bus* ads.

Researchers cautioned, however, that direct causal connections cannot be established; the results of ad effectiveness evaluations based on ad recall may be compromised by differences in the attitudes of those who are able to recall the ads. For example, those who already have strong anti-smoking attitudes may pay more attention to the ads regardless of the specific message content (Farrelly et al., 2002).

U.S./California

The California Department of Health Services Tobacco Control Section has aired tobacco industry deceptive-practices ads for more than a decade. Many researchers in that state and elsewhere believe that these types of ads played a role, as did other messages, in contributing to the decline in youth smoking prevalence in the state among those aged 12–17 years, from 8.7% in 1992 to 5.9% in 2001 (Balbach and Glantz, 1998; Goldman and Glantz, 1998). In a review of broadcast messages from 1994 to 2000, the Independent Evaluation Consortium for the State of California Department of Health Services Tobacco Control Section found that 40% of these ads focused on prevention and cessation, 32% on tobacco industry deceptive practices, and 22% on secondhand smoke (Independent Evaluation Consortium, April 2003).

This study found that youth and adults who had seen more of the California campaign's tobacco counter-marketing television ads emphasizing the deceptive practices of tobacco companies were more likely to believe that tobacco advertising and promotions influence youth to smoke (Independent Evaluation Consortium, 1998). The evaluation of four television ads showed that ads focusing on the harm caused to others by tobacco use and exposing tobacco industry deceptive practices had the highest combination of recall and accuracy of recall (the ability to correctly describe the ad). Ads with the highest scores for both recall and accuracy of recall among youth were *Victim/Wife*, which featured a man whose wife had died from an illness caused by his cigarette smoke, and *Hooked*, which suggested that tobacco companies use addiction to achieve their business goals.

U.S./Florida

The Florida state tobacco control program first developed the Truth campaign concept, later adopted by the American Legacy Foundation, in which a series of ads inform youth about tobacco industry deceptive marketing practices. Florida's youth-targeted anti-smoking campaign included grassroots activism, public relations activities, school-based programs, and a strong mass media presence.

From 1998 to 2000, when the campaign received strong funding support from the state legislature through the Florida Department of Health, cigarette smoking among middle school students dropped from 18.5% to 11.1% (a relative decline of 40%) and among high school students from 27.4% to 22.6% (a relative decline of 18%) (Bauer and Johnson, 2001).

The Florida Anti-Tobacco Media Evaluation (FAME) found that the more tobacco industry deceptive-practices ads Florida teens, especially younger teens, saw during the campaign, the less likely they were to begin smoking (Sly et al., 2001). The FAME longitudinal study assessed recall of specific tobacco counter-marketing ads in Florida's Truth campaign and actual changes in smoking behavior. Confirmed awareness of the Truth advertising campaign correlated strongly with reduced likelihood of becoming a smoker and with increased likelihood of quitting. Teens who agreed strongly with statements about tobacco industry deceptive practices had smoking initiation rates that were 7.3 times lower than those of teens who agreed less strongly with the statements, and more than two times lower than those of teens with medium levels of agreement (Sly et al., 2001).

A direct causal relationship between reported ad exposure and smoking prevalence, initiation, or cessation cannot be confirmed because of selective recall and pre-existing attitudes. The ads were part of a larger effort to reduce smoking, making it difficult to determine which component of the tobacco counter-marketing effort had the greatest influence on smoking initiation rates. Nevertheless, the reductions in smoking prevalence were extremely impressive, especially given the short duration of the campaign (Sly et al., 2001).

Table 8

Beliefs Among Teens in U.S./Florida and in a U.S./National Sample Regarding Tobacco Industry Behavior

Belief Statement	% of Florida Teens in Agreement	% of Teens Nationally in Agreement
Cigarette companies lie.	87.3	81.5
Cigarette companies deny that cigarettes cause cancer.	65.9	56.8
Cigarette companies try to get teens to start smoking.	88.1	82.1
I would like to see cigarette companies go out of business.	83.3	77.1

Value differences between Florida teens and the national sample were statistically significant based on nonoverlapping 95% confidence intervals. (RTI International, 2002)

The FAME findings regarding the effectiveness of tobacco industry deceptive-practices ads on youth in Florida were confirmed by the American Legacy Media Tracking Surveys, which gauged the effectiveness of the national truth[sm] campaign (RTI International, 2002). The LMTS included a relatively large number of participants in Florida to allow assessment of the incremental effect of the in-state Truth campaign. The researchers found that Florida teens were more likely to have unfavorable beliefs about the tobacco industry than their peers in other parts of the country, possibly because they had been exposed to the messages of both campaigns and to the tobacco industry deceptive-practices theme for a longer period of time (Table 8).

U.S./Minnesota

Beginning in 1999, the Minnesota Department of Health initiated the Target Market campaign to increase knowledge and levels of emotion about tobacco industry deceptive practices by educating Minnesota youth about the industry and encouraging them to join a youth anti-tobacco movement. The campaign included ads featuring youth speaking out against the tobacco industry that had targeted them as potential consumers.

After 1 year of the campaign, the Minnesota Target Market campaign evaluation indicated that the Target Market message had affected smoking behavior and teen attitudes about the tobacco industry. Youth aged 12–13 years showed the most growth in confidence in their ability to fight back against tobacco industry messages that encourage smoking, along with a new level of interest in, and enhanced knowledge of, tobacco industry deceptive practices (Table 9) (Ergo International, 2001).

Minnesota youth also reported changes in smoking behavior and anti-tobacco beliefs following the Target Market campaign's first year (Table 10). In the 2001 Target Market campaign evaluation study, the number of Minnesota youth who reported using tobacco in the last 21 days dropped from 3% to 1% among those aged 12–13 years, and from 30% to 23% among those aged 16–17 years. These declines were statistically significant (Ergo International, 2001).

Table 9

Beliefs About the U.S./Minnesota Target Market (TM) Advertising Messages Among Youth Who Recalled Seeing or Hearing TM Ad(s)

	Youth Responses (%)		
Belief Statements	12- to 13-year-olds Before/After Campaign	14- to 15-year-olds Before/After Campaign	16- to 17-year-olds Before/After Campaign
Like you have the power to fight back	80/92	80/86	79/82*
That you learned something new	54/73	47/67	33/63
Motivated you	48/65	41/57	37/57
Inspired you	47/68	37/58	23/51

* All differences in values pre-campaign and post-campaign (before and after viewing the ads) were statistically significant based on nonoverlapping 95% confidence intervals, except for the belief statement "Like you have the power to fight back" for 16- to 17-year-olds. Numbers in parentheses indicate numbers of participants in each cell. (Ergo International, 2001)

Table 10

Changes in Anti-Tobacco Beliefs Associated with the Mass Media Campaign Among U.S./Minnesota Youth Aged 12–17 Years

Belief Statements	Youth Response (%)	
	Before seeing the ads	After seeing the ads
I don't want to be the target of big tobacco companies.	71	76
I feel strongly against smoking.	69	75
It annoys me that tobacco companies are targeting kids.	57	63
Knowing how much money tobacco companies are making off of kids makes me mad.	56	63
Cigarette companies are trying to get young people to smoke.	52	66
Cigarette companies try to cover up all of the bad things they have done.	48	55
I can fight back against tobacco companies.	42	57
It doesn't matter to me if other kids smoke or not.	22	19

All differences were significant at the 95% confidence level. (Ergo International, 2001)

Target Market annual funding was reduced from $23.7 million to $4.6 million in 2003, eliminating all broadcast presence (CDC, 2004). Within 6 months of the reduced media presence, the percentage of adolescents who reported susceptibility to smoking increased from 43% to 53%.

Message Research

Canada/British Columbia

In British Columbia, students who participated in the Critics' Choice school program found tobacco industry deceptive-practices ads difficult to understand and uninteresting (British Columbia Ministry of Health, 2000). Ads that included a tobacco industry message were not rated in the top 5 or 6 of the 12 ads viewed each year, based on youth perceptions of the ads' ability to encourage cessation or discourage smoking initiation. The exception was *Body Bags*, ranked second in 2000, which reported the number of deaths caused annually by tobacco-related diseases and used graphic visuals of body bags (British Columbia Ministry of Health, 2000). The strong response to *Body Bags* may indicate the value of blending a health-effects message with a tobacco industry deceptive-practices message.

A consultant to the British Columbia Ministry of Health's advertising agency that managed the Critics' Choice program proposed that the lack of positive response to the tobacco industry deceptive-practices ads was probably due to two factors (Kim Sanderson, unpublished data, June 2001):

- The cigarette brand names used in the ads, such as Marlboro, and company names, such Philip Morris, were not very familiar to Canadian youth because these brands and companies' products were not sold in that part of Canada.

- Because of tobacco advertising restrictions, the tobacco industry's presence was less prominent in Canada than in other countries.

U.S./Multistate
In 1999, CDC sponsored a multistate focus groups study in Massachusetts, California, and Arizona. Tobacco industry deceptive-practices messages were better understood and received among respondents who lived in states where these messages had already been communicated extensively, such as California. Youth in states where tobacco industry deceptive-practices messages had not been extensively aired did not understand the ads and lacked interest in them (Teen Research Unlimited, 1999).

U.S./California
To review the effectiveness of anti-smoking television ads developed or in development for youth and adults, researchers at the University of California, San Francisco conducted a national anti-smoking campaign focus group analysis. They studied results from 186 focus groups that evaluated eight advertising themes (industry deceptive practices, secondhand smoke, addiction, cessation, youth access, short-term effects, long-term health effects, and romantic rejection). The researchers concluded that tobacco industry deceptive-practices and secondhand-smoke messages were the most effective for de-normalizing smoking and reducing cigarette consumption (Goldman and Glantz, 1998). Other researchers, however, took issue with the findings of this study, noting that because of methodological limitations, the research did not necessarily support these conclusions (Worden et al., 1998; Balch and Rudham, 1998).

The University of California, Irvine Protection Motivation Theory Message Study investigated several types of approaches used in tobacco industry deceptive-practices ads with students in middle and high school. The students compared these ads, which included a range of messages such as tobacco industry marketing tactics, deaths caused by such tactics, and youth activism against tobacco marketers. None of the tobacco industry deceptive-practices approaches were found to lessen youths' intent to smoke. Respondents did, however, have favorable opinions about the ads, and the ads increased their knowledge about tobacco industry marketing (Pechmann et al., 2003).

U.S./North Carolina
In the North Carolina anti-smoking ads focus groups conducted among students living in this tobacco-growing state, ads with a tobacco industry deceptive-practices theme were rated considerably lower than ads with other themes in their ability to cause the viewer to stop and think about tobacco use. The students who gave low ratings to the industry deceptive-practices ads commented that the decision whether to smoke is up to youth, and the tobacco industry has a very limited impact on youth decisions. Others noted that tobacco companies have a right to make money. Participants rated the ads with a tobacco industry deceptive-practices message as more effective in making them stop and think when the ads included health risk information (University of North Carolina, 2001).

Social Approval/Disapproval or Refusal Skills

Mass Media Campaign Evaluations

The Netherlands
The Netherlands DEFACTO campaign conducted from 1998 to 2000 included mass media (television and radio ads and publicity about the campaign), a road show, a Web site, and cessation services (Frissen, 2002). The objective of the campaign was to decrease smoking and exposure to secondhand smoke in Dutch society. The ads showed that youth do not need to smoke to be independent and popular and that non-smokers are cool.

The television ads featured obnoxious, rebellious behavior, such as burping in a classroom, as a way to express the coolness of a nonsmoker. The Netherlands DEFACTO tracking study, conducted 10 weeks after the campaign began, found that 72% of those surveyed understood the ads and 71% appreciated them (Frissen, 2002). The percentage of youth who had strong intentions to continue not to smoke increased from 32% to 42% during this campaign. Those who had weaker intentions to continue not to smoke decreased from 42% to 33%. During this period, the percentage of youth who reported that they did not have smoking friends increased from 17% to 23% (Frissen, 2002).

U.S./Vermont, Montana, New York

In 1986, researchers at the University of Vermont began a multistate combined school and mass media study, developing television ads that reached youth in grades 5–10 with social-disapproval, refusal-skills, and smoking-consequences messages (Flynn et al., 1995). The ads were developed based on feedback from focus groups, testing of creative ideas, and reviews of completed ads by the target audiences to help ensure that the ads would provide youth with a positive view of not smoking, a negative view of smoking, improved skills for refusing cigarettes, and a clearer understanding that most youth their age do not smoke. These researchers did not develop or test ads with messages about the long-term health effects of smoking or tobacco industry deceptive-practices messages for comparison. The ads were broadcast on television in Vermont, Montana, and south central New York State communities.

The researchers measured the impact of a mass media campaign in conjunction with a typical school tobacco use prevention program. Students who participated in the school program and saw the ads smoked fewer cigarettes per week (2.6) following the campaign than students who participated only in the school program (4.4). Moreover, only 13% of students who participated in the school program and saw the ads had smoked a cigarette in the previous week, compared with 20% of those who participated in the school program only (Flynn et al., 1995). The reductions in smoking prevalence among youth exposed to the campaign lasted up to 2 years after the campaign had stopped. The multistate school mass media campaign follow-up study calculated that the odds ratio for being a weekly smoker after exposure to both mass media and school-based programs was 0.6, indicating a reduced risk (Flynn et al., 1994).

U.S./Minnesota

The Minnesota Department of Health developed and implemented a comprehensive tobacco counter-marketing campaign from 1986 to 1990 designed to discourage tobacco use among schoolchildren (Murray et al., 1994). Annual spending for the mass media portion of the campaign was about $2 million. The campaign used a social approval-disapproval and refusal-skills approach. The campaign developers sought to present not smoking in a positive light and smoking as negative behavior, and to provide training on how to refuse invitations to smoke.

The campaign was evaluated annually through the Minnesota-Wisconsin Adolescent Tobacco Use Research Project. Evaluation results based on Arbitron data, which measure household television viewing patterns, indicate that while the target audience was aware of the messages (95% of the 3,600 9th-grade students surveyed annually had seen an anti-smoking message at least 50 times per year), no measurable changes in attitudes or smoking behavior occurred as a result of the 4-year campaign. Researchers believe that the lack of change may have been due to less than full support of schools in providing a strong anti-smoking curriculum (Murray et al., 1994).

Message Research

U.S./California

The University of California, Irvine Protection Motivation Theory Message Study found that the ads students rated as most likely to strengthen their intentions not to smoke addressed social-norms themes, conveying that smoking may cause severe social disapproval by peers. Anti-smoking messages rated as effective in increasing youth intentions not to smoke, compared with control-group messages that focused on drunk driving, discussed smokers' negative life circumstances (disheveled "losers" who had taken the wrong path in life and as a result had unattractive life situations), role modeling to enhance viewers' refusal skills, and information on how smoking endangers the lives of others. The perceived lack of appeal of smoking due to the severity of social disapproval risks appeared to have the greatest effect on students' intentions not to smoke. Message themes that were rated as less effective included disease and death (health effects), cosmetics (effects of smoking on appearance, such as bad breath), selling disease and death (tobacco companies influencing consumers to purchase products that cause illness and death), and tobacco industry marketing tactics (powerful tobacco companies targeting children, women, and minorities) (Pechmann et al., 2003).

U.S./Massachusetts

The Massachusetts tobacco surveys measured recall and perceived effectiveness of eight ads used in the

Massachusetts Department of Health tobacco control media campaign. The lowest recall rate was for ads in the normative category, which delivered messages about social approval of not smoking and disapproval of smoking (Biener, 2004).

Secondhand Smoke

Mass Media Campaign Evaluations

U.S./California

Since 1993, reducing secondhand-smoke exposure has been one of the major goals of the California tobacco control program. The California Independent Evaluation Research Consortium conducted surveys from 1989 to 1995 to evaluate many aspects of the California state tobacco control program and to provide information on which media ads were most highly associated with attitude changes. Exposure to secondhand-smoke messages was associated with an increase in the number of adults and youth who believed that breathing secondhand smoke was bad for one's health, and an increase in the likelihood of respondents asking another person not to smoke around them (Independent Evaluation Consortium, 1998) (Table 12).

The Independent Evaluation Consortium found that the *Victim Wife* ad, which featured a man whose wife had died from extensive exposure to secondhand smoke, achieved the highest recall and accuracy of recall of any ad in the study for both adults and youth (Independent Evaluation Consortium, 1998).

A review of all messages broadcast in California from 1994 to 2000 found that 22% of the television spots aired addressed concerns about secondhand smoke, 40% focused on prevention and cessation, and 32% provided information on tobacco industry deceptive practices (Independent Evaluation Consortium, 2003). Smoking prevalence among California youth remained flat at 11.2% from 1994 to 1997, followed by a large 1-year decline of 10.7% to 6.9% from 1998 to 1999. This decrease corresponded with a significant increase in media campaign spending, from $13.3 million in 1998 to $19.5 million in 1999. The decline in California youth smoking prevalence continued, dropping to 5.9% in 2001 (California Youth Tobacco Survey, 2002).

Table 12

Effect of Viewing U.S./California Secondhand Smoke Messages on Beliefs and Behaviors

	Number of Secondhand-Smoke Ads Viewed					
	None		1–2		2+	
Belief/Behavior	10th-Grade Youth (%)	Adults (%)	10th-Grade Youth (%)	Adults (%)	10th-Grade Youth (%)	Adults (%)
Believe that secondhand smoke is a health risk	92	87	97	91	100	93
Likely to ask someone not to smoke around them	41	38	47	42	48	48

(Independent Evaluation Consortium, 1998)

Canada/Ontario

The Ontario, Canada, Ministry of Health launched a media campaign to communicate the dangers of secondhand smoke. The campaign was designed to reduce the social acceptability of smoking in public places and to affect public policy by communicating the health risks of secondhand smoke to nonsmokers. Television advertising that addressed the health risks of secondhand smoke succeeded in raising awareness and interest in the topic (Lacey, 2002). The post-campaign Ontario tobacco media campaign tracking survey showed that awareness of the *Victim/Wife* ad was slightly higher for youth (81%) than for adults (76%), and that 96% of youth believed that second-hand smoke was a danger to others besides smokers. Overall, youth tended to hold similar views about secondhand smoke to those of the adults, but were more accepting of smokers in social situations. Youth were supportive of government regulations to control smoking in public places (87%, compared with 85% of adults) and more likely than adults to agree that smoking should be illegal (56%, compared with 49% of adults) (Lacey, 2002).

Message Research

U.S./California, U.S./Massachusetts, U.S./Michigan

The University of California, San Francisco's national anti-smoking advertising campaign focus-group analyses found that secondhand smoke and tobacco industry deceptive practices were the two most effective message themes of the eight tested for de-normalizing smoking and reducing cigarette consumption (Goldman and Glantz, 1998). However, as mentioned earlier, this study's methods and assumptions were questioned by some members of the tobacco control community (Balch and Rudham, 1998; Worden et al., 1998).

U.S./California

The University of California, Irvine Protection Motivation Theory Message Study found that ads that discussed the negative effects of smoking and secondhand smoke on family members and other people weakened youths' intent to smoke. In particular, students rated the perceived effectiveness of secondhand-smoke ad messages as higher than that of messages concerning health risks to smokers or tobacco industry deceptive practices (Pechmann et al., 2003). According to the authors, the ads worked because they implied that people do not appreciate living or working with smokers, or they see the behavior as inconsiderate, harmful to them, and socially unacceptable.

U.S./North Carolina

Youth participants in the North Carolina Anti-smoking Ads Focus Groups study rated secondhand-smoke messages as the second most effective theme of those tested, with only messages on adverse health effects to smokers rated higher. Participants indicated that ads using this theme raised awareness of the dangers of secondhand smoke, which appeared to be new information to some participants (University of North Carolina, 2002).

Cosmetic Effects

Mass Media Campaign Evaluations

U.S./Arizona

The Arizona TEPP ad campaign included a focus on the short-term effects of smoking on a teen's breath, teeth, and skin, and how these effects can interfere with a teen's desired appearance. With a tagline of "Tobacco. Tumor causing, teeth staining, smelly puking habit," these ads presented a range of unattractive and humorous scenarios, often exaggerating the effects of tobacco on the health, appearance, and social acceptance of youth who smoke.

The in-school evaluation of the Arizona TEPP prevention ads studied youth response to the television ads used in 1999 to determine which emotions were most influential in generating disapproval of smoking and the intention not to smoke. The research showed that the most effective ads tested among Arizona youth were those rated as the most disgusting (i.e., generating a negative emotional response); messages of social disapproval were rated as less effective (Hendricks et al., 2001). Researchers tested reactions to ads created and used in Arizona only and did not examine the impact of any of the graphic health-effects or testimonial ads that have been shown to be effective elsewhere.

U.S./Massachusetts

The Massachusetts tobacco surveys of high school students evaluated the effectiveness of various ad executions. The researchers found that ads presenting the impact of cigarette smoking on appearance were more effective than ads using humor, in that more youth were able to recall the appearance-focused ads and were more receptive to the messages. However, these ads were less effective than those described as sad or frightening by youth respondents (Biener, 2002).

Message Research

U.S./California

The University of California, Irvine Protection Motivation Theory Message Study of school-based groups found that ads showing the effects of smoking on appearance and attractiveness (e.g., bad breath, yellowed teeth, smelly clothes) did not influence respondents' intentions to smoke, apparently because the youth felt that appearance problems could be easily remedied with cosmetic products (Pechmann et al., 2003).

Addiction

Message Research

U.S./Multistate

Most young people do not understand the addictive characteristics of tobacco use and mistakenly believe that they can quit using tobacco whenever they please (CDC, 1994). However, smoking cessation is much harder than most youth perceive it to be (CDC, 2001). Creating messages about the power of nicotine addiction that are comprehensible and relevant to the viewer is difficult. One of the most powerful ads addressing addiction (along with health effects) is the *Debi/Voice Box* ad. However, the TRU multistate focus group research indicated that youth audiences named health effects, not addiction, as the main message of the *Debi* ad (Teenage Research Unlimited, 1999).

U.S./Massachusetts

According to an account executive from the advertising agency that developed the U.S./Massachusetts tobacco counter-marketing campaign, the program's efforts to communicate messages about addiction using the testimonial format did not achieve the impact of testimonials portraying illness and personal loss (Miller, unpublished data, 2000). In one set of Massachusetts ads, teenagers talked remorsefully about how they wished they had never started to smoke. These ads did not achieve nearly the awareness and recall ratings of the personal-loss ads.

Another Massachusetts ad that attempted to communicate the power of addiction was the *Breathe* ad. It featured a swimmer underwater needing to take a breath in an attempt to compare the need for a cigarette to the basic need to breathe. Many Massachusetts youth did not understand the connection to smoking (Miller, oral communication, October 2000).

Athletic Performance

Mass Media Campaign Evaluations

U.S./National

The Philip Morris *Karate Kid* ad, which was designed to communicate the message that smoking causes shortness of breath and can affect athletic performance, was evaluated in the Legacy Media Tracking Surveys (LMTS) for awareness and receptivity compared with the American Legacy Foundation's ads addressing health effects or tobacco industry deceptive practices. The *Karate Kid* ad received a lower rating than any of the Legacy ads reviewed (See Table 7) (Farrelly et al., 2002).

U.S./Massachusetts

The *Models* ad, which featured members of the U.S. women's Olympic soccer team, was one of eight ads from the Massachusetts Department of Health tobacco control media campaign evaluated for emotional tone and message content through Massachusetts tobacco surveys with Massachusetts youth aged 12–17 years. In the ad, the soccer players talked about being able to perform better in sports because they did not smoke. The ad received lower ratings for recall and effectiveness than health-effects messages and humorous messages aired in the Massachusetts campaign and tested in the research (Biener, 2004).

Message Research

U.S./National

The 1998 CDC-sponsored National Quantitative Copy Test compared recall among youth audiences of the *Cowboy* ad, which addressed the serious negative health effects of smoking, with the *Models* ad, in which members of the U.S. women's soccer team talked about being able to perform better in sports by not smoking. The *Models* ad featured a celebrity role model cautioning the audience about tobacco industry messages glamorizing smoking, versus the reality of the effects of smoking on athletic performance. Recall of the *Models* ad was below average compared with hundreds of other consumer product ads tested, in both ability to recall seeing the ad 3 days after the first research interview and being able to recall the main message of the ad. Only 19% of respondents could recall a key element of the ad, and only 8% of female respondents aged 13–19 could state that the message of the ad was about improving athletic performance by not smoking (Gutierrez, personal communication, 1998).

Individual Choice

Mass Media Campaign Evaluations

U.S./National

Most tobacco industry-sponsored, youth-focused ads have stressed individual-choice messages, emphasizing that youth can make decisions independently about whether to smoke, and encouraging them to choose not to smoke. The Philip Morris ad campaign, which focused on individual choice, was launched in 1998, with annual spending reported to be in excess of $100 million for mass media alone. This media expenditure was substantially higher than that of the American Legacy Foundation for its ad placement campaign (Farrelly et al., 2002).

When the Legacy ads were compared with the Philip Morris individual-choice ads in the Legacy Media Tracking Study, the individual-choice ads were rated as less effective than the Legacy ads in building awareness and being positively received by the target audiences. Nearly 75% of respondents could confirm awareness of at least one Legacy ad, versus 66% of any Philip Morris individual-choice ad (Farrelly et al., 2002).

Analysis of the LMTS data allowed comparisons of the Legacy ads to individual-choice ads produced by Philip Morris and Lorillard (Tobacco Is Whacko campaign), all of which aired in 2000. Results showed that the industry-sponsored ads were significantly less well received by youth who were current smokers or most susceptible to smoking (based on the number of friends and family members who smoked and their attitudes toward tobacco and tobacco companies). Of the five message types tested, the ads combining tobacco industry deceptive-practices messages with health-risk information received the highest receptivity ratings among youth and young adults. The recall numbers are especially striking because respondents were six times more likely to remember the Legacy ads than the tobacco industry ads (Farrelly et al., 2002).

Message Research

Scotland

The Center for Tobacco Control Research at the University of Strathclyde conducted focus groups among respondents aged 12–17 in Scotland in November 2001 to determine youth reactions to the tobacco industry-sponsored Youth Smoking Prevention (YSP) ads aired on MTV (Devlin et al., 2002). Results from the Scotland YSP ads focus groups indicated that ads emphasizing individual choice did not help persuade youth participants not to smoke. In addition, the youth failed to relate to the campaign, feeling that the messages were not relevant to their lives. Participants described the television ads as unrealistic and lacking credibility. In addition, the campaign ads appeared to reinforce young smokers' decisions to smoke by implying that both smoking and not smoking were acceptable, and the ads did not address any serious negative consequences of tobacco use (Devlin et al., 2002).

U.S./Multistate

The TRU multistate focus groups study addressed several individual-choice ads, including the *Stairs* and *Bus* ads from Philip Morris and the *I Decide* ad from U.S./Arizona. The ads that focused on individual choice (i.e., encouraged viewers to make their own decisions about smoking or stated that one does not need to smoke to be cool) were consistently rated lowest by participants in their likelihood of making participants "stop and think about not using tobacco." Participants stated that the ads did not have enough substance because they did not include good reasons not to smoke and did not provide any compelling information about the consequences of smoking (Teenage Research Unlimited, 1999).

U.S./California

The University of California, Irvine Protection Motivation Theory Message Testing study was designed, in part, to examine the effects of the Philip Morris Think. Don't Smoke. campaign individual-choice ads. The researchers found that these ads did not have any effect on youth intentions to smoke (Pechmann et al.,

2003). According to the researchers, many of the Philip Morris ads seemed to imply that both smoking and not smoking are socially acceptable choices, which does not constitute a clear anti-smoking message.

Effectiveness of Different Message Themes

Based on our review of ad themes and media campaigns stressing each of these themes, we have classified the effectiveness of each message theme into one of four categories: effective, effective but with limited research data, inconclusive, or not effective.

Effective: Health Effects

Media campaign and message evaluation research has consistently shown that portraying the serious negative consequences of smoking in a credible manner is effective in influencing youth; in some instances, these messages were shown to have a positive influence on attitudes or behaviors concerning not using tobacco. Adult-targeted messages that portray personal loss and present information on health risks that was not previously known or previously considered can be effective among youth, even when the messages are not targeted to youth audiences (Hassard, 2000). These findings about the power of new health information in reaching audiences effectively are consistent with those from a meta-analysis of 48 health campaigns in the United States (Snyder, 2001). In that study, researchers found that the most effective campaigns were those that provided the audience with new information (not previously considered or known) on health effects.

Simply presenting health information is not enough. New information or new perspectives need to be presented in ways that engage viewers emotionally. For example, the Australian Every Cigarette Is Doing You Damage ads and the *Janet Sackman, Cowboy, Voice-Box/Debi*, and *Doesn't Kill* ads from the United States demonstrate the importance of health-effects message content delivered in formats that are engaging to viewers (e.g., graphic display of health effects, testimonials about personal loss and suffering) (University of Arizona, 2000; Biener, 2002; Hassard, 2000; Murphy, 2000; Teenage Research Unlimited, 1999).

Effective: Tobacco Industry Deceptive Practices

The effectiveness of messages in a mass media campaign emphasizing the deceptive practices of the tobacco industry has been assessed mainly in the United States. Effectiveness of this approach in other countries is not known. Many, but not all, of the studies on these ads found that tobacco industry deceptive-practices ads can successfully influence youth knowledge about the tobacco industry, attitudes toward smoking and the tobacco industry and, in some cases, smoking behaviors. Combining messages about the deceptive practices of the tobacco industry with health-effects messages has been shown to be effective in changing youth attitudes and influencing behaviors (Balbach and Glantz, 1998; Independent Evaluation Consortium, 1998).

The youth-focused tobacco industry deceptive-practices message strategy requires audience preparation and may be misunderstood by audiences unfamiliar with tobacco industry strategies and behaviors. Youth audiences may need a clear explanation of why the tobacco industry should be viewed differently than other legal businesses, and they probably need exposure to many different messages over time to fully understand this relatively complex subject.

Effective but with Limited Research Data: Social Approval/Disapproval or Refusal Skills

Messages addressing social approval of not smoking or social disapproval of smoking or that introduce refusal skills have been found in some studies to be effective in increasing awareness of tobacco prevention issues among youth and reducing intentions to smoke. One study found that when such ads are used in conjunction with a school-based educational intervention, they contribute to a decline in smoking prevalence (Flynn et al., 1995). Ads that communicate the social approval or disapproval theme or refusal skills have been effective in changing attitudes and behavior in different countries. However, the number of evaluations available for this review was small and results available from one large-scale broadcast campaign evaluation did not indicate that this message strategy was effective in changing attitudes or behavior, even though the audience was aware of the messages (Murray et al., 1994). As a result, we classified these ads as effective in limited controlled research environments.

Effective but with Limited Research Data: Secondhand Smoke

Research results on the effectiveness of secondhand-smoke message content are positive, but the secondhand-smoke message has rarely been used as a sole or major focus in a youth tobacco use prevention campaign. As a result, data on this theme are very limited.

Inconclusive: Cosmetic and Short-Term Effects

Findings on cosmetic and short-term–effect ads were available for this review from only three studies conducted in the United States, and results were inconclusive. Additional research is needed before any conclusion can be reached about the effectiveness of this type of message content.

Inconclusive: Addiction

Research on this type of message content is limited. However, the results that are available suggest that this theme is less effective among youth than other message themes.

Inconclusive: Athletic Performance

Research on this type of message content is limited. However, the results that are available suggest that messages with this theme are less effective among youth than other message themes.

Not Effective: Individual Choice

Research indicates that the individual-choice message is not effective in preventing youth from using tobacco.

MESSAGE FORMAT

Message format refers to the method or creative approach used to present message content to audiences. Although many formats have been used in tobacco use prevention ads, research data and campaign lessons compiled for this review focus on the three most commonly used:

- Testimonials—real people speaking about their losses, pain, and suffering due to the consequences of smoking.

- Graphic depiction—visual images showing the adverse health effects of smoking in novel, credible ways.

- Celebrities—well-known people from the entertainment, sports, or political fields presenting anti-tobacco messages.

Testimonials

England
The *Stephen* and *Rebecca* testimonial ads evaluated in the England anti-smoking ad tracking survey received higher agreement among youth than adults that older people are not the only ones who suffer from smoking-related illnesses and that continuing to try to quit is important regardless of age (BMRB Social Research, 2002).

U.S./Massachusetts
A representative from Arnold Communications, the advertising agency that created the Massachusetts *Pam Laffin* and *Rick Stoddard* testimonial ad series, noted in an internal agency memo that real-life stories tend to resonate across multiple target audiences (Brogdon, oral communication, 2000). The agency learned through conversations with youth that the *Pam Laffin* ads, originally targeted to adult smokers, seemed to resonate well with teens because of Pam's own youth and the startling photos in the ad of Pam before and after she developed emphysema.

The *Pam Laffin* pre- and post-campaign telephone surveys for the Massachusetts 1997 ad tracking study found that 94% of youth aged 9–17 years who recalled the ad believed that it provided good reasons not to smoke. When responses from youth who had seen the ad were compared with responses from youth who could not recall seeing the ad, 16% more youth who had seen the ad reported believing that "smoking was not a way to look cool," and 12% more agreed that "smoking was not a way to look and feel independent" (Massachusetts Department of Public Health, 1997).

In the *Janet Sackman* ad, a former cigarette ad model who has lost her vocal cords to cancer describes the addictiveness of smoking and how she was misled by the tobacco companies she had once worked for as a highly visible spokeswoman. Massachusetts youth rated this ad as effective in evoking strong negative emotions about the effects of smoking in the Massachusetts Tobacco Surveys and longitudinal studies. Youth described this ad as sad and frightening, and they considered ads that evoke such emotions to be more effective than ads rated as funny or neutral (Biener, 2004).

U.S./Arizona
In the *Doesn't Kill* ad, teenagers report that their parents and friends had been told that tobacco would kill them, but this did not happen. When their parents' and friends' faces are revealed, the viewer sees their current health conditions caused by smoking-related diseases; for example, one father's jaw and cheek have been removed, one mother has a stoma in her throat resulting from losing part of her larynx, and part of

another woman's mouth is missing. The Arizona TEPP media campaign evaluation results indicated that youth were more likely to remember the *Doesn't Kill* ad than other ads reviewed in the research. In addition, significantly more respondents agreed that the *Doesn't Kill* ad would make teenagers think about quitting smoking than any of the other ads or groups of ads (University of Arizona, 2000).

U.S./Multistate

The TRU multistate and University of North Carolina focus group studies found that ads that graphically, dramatically, and emotionally portrayed the serious negative consequences of smoking were rated as the most effective by participants in making them "stop and think about not using tobacco." Three of the four most highly rated ads (*Voicebox/Debi, Pam Laffin,* and *Cowboy*) used a testimonial format to deliver their messages. The real stories of personal loss and the impact on the smokers' families were messages that youth reported identifying with, in part because virtually all of them knew someone who had died or suffered from a tobacco-related disease. Participants who had seen the ads also claimed that they would never want to be like the smokers in the ads who suffered physically from tobacco (Teenage Research Unlimited, 1999; University of North Carolina, 2001).

U.S./Utah

The Utah Department of Health tobacco media campaign formative message research demonstrated that, of all the ads tested, testimonial-format ads illustrating the suffering caused by the health effects of using tobacco were most likely to interest and persuade youth (Neiger et al., 2002).

Graphic Depiction

Australia

The developers of the Australian Every Cigarette is Doing You Damage campaign found new ways to show audiences exactly what cigarette smoking can do to the human body. The ads showed how tobacco-related diseases develop, presenting the viewer with previously unknown information about the health effects of smoking. The Australia national tobacco campaign surveys showed that the *Artery* ad achieved a higher rate of youth recall (73%) than the *Lung* ad (60%), which conveyed a message about a health risk, lung damage, with which smokers are more familiar. The *Tumour* ad, which showed how smoking can damage cells and lead to tumor growth, also achieved higher recall (64%) than the *Lung* ad (Hassard, 2000).

U.S./Arizona

The Arizona prevention ads in-school evaluation was designed to evaluate the appeal and impact of emotion in anti-tobacco ad messages. The researchers tested a variety of ads that had been used in the state's youth-targeted tobacco counter-advertising campaign. The ads were rated for their ability to elicit emotional reactions of disgust, humor, fear, and guilt. Ads rated as disgusting were perceived as most effective in causing these reactions; these ads had a strong element of graphic display, such as the repulsive characteristics of spit tobacco juice (Hendricks et al., 2001).

Celebrities

U.S./National

The CDC-sponsored National Quantitative Copy Test compared two ads, *Models* and *Cowboy*, that featured celebrities. The *Models* ad, which featured the women's U.S. Olympic soccer team, had low recall among the target audience of females aged 13–19 years. The testimonial ad *Cowboy*, which shows the suffering from smoking-related disease of the actor who played the Marlboro Man, had much higher recall levels than the *Models* ad across all audiences tested. The researchers believed that this was because the ad evoked more emotion and presented realistic, negative consequences of smoking (Gutierrez, personal communication, 1998).

Celebrities can help build awareness by generating media coverage at events and news conferences (Zollo, 1999). In addition, celebrities can attract the attention of policy makers to the importance of youth tobacco use prevention.

Celebrity personal testimonial ads involve both a testimonial and a celebrity format. Examples of ads using celebrities include ads featuring U.S. supermodel Christy Turlington, who quit smoking after many attempts and who lost her father to lung cancer caused by smoking, and Rick Bender, a U.S. semi-professional baseball player whose jaw and cheek were removed because of cancer caused by chewing tobacco.

The most credible celebrity spokespeople for tobacco counter-advertising messages seem to be those who have experienced firsthand the effects of tobacco use, such as former smokers who speak from experience about the negative health consequences of smoking or the difficulty of quitting or who have lost a family member because of tobacco use.

Several potential concerns must be considered before using celebrities as spokespeople in youth counter-marketing campaigns. Youth are media savvy and highly aware that celebrities are often paid to tout product messages, potentially compromising celebrities' credibility (Zollo, 1999). In addition, some program managers have found that in their desire to be involved in the development of the advertising, celebrities may overestimate their value and influence and may direct a campaign's communication in ways that are not supported by best practices. Furthermore, a campaign may lose its credibility if a celebrity smoker who quits begins using tobacco again, abuses another substance (such as drugs or alcohol), or becomes involved in a scandal (Johnson, 1992; Zollo, 1999).

Several campaigns have benefited when people who were not famous presented personal testimonies in anti-tobacco ads and *became* celebrities in their hometowns, states, or countries. Pam Laffin, a U.S./Massachusetts spokeswoman who suffered from smoking-related illnesses, talked to youth audiences around that state, testified at legislative hearings in several states, and was featured in an MTV documentary before her death in October 2001. Debi Austin, the smoker who lost her voice box to cancer, was asked to carry the Olympic torch in her home state of California.

Conclusions

Good evidence indicates that testimonials are an effective ad format for youth. They provide a strong emotional appeal because they are based on stories of real people who have suffered from the consequences of their tobacco use or the tobacco use of loved ones. This finding is consistent with an extensive body of research in communication, psychology, and advertising about the impact of testimonial messages on audiences (Dillard and Pfau, 2002; Slater, 2002).

Although less research is available on their effectiveness, graphic depictions of the health effects of smoking also are an effective format with youth audiences. As with testimonials, strong graphic displays can induce strong negative emotional reactions (e.g., disgust, fear), which probably contributes to their effectiveness. Graphic displays, however, must be credible and based on health information that was previously unknown or unconsidered to influence viewers.

Quantitative evaluation data are lacking, but program managers have learned that celebrities can increase awareness of a campaign message. This format must be used with caution, however, because credibility concerns and unexpected revelations of celebrity misdeeds can damage the effectiveness of ad campaigns using celebrities (Zollo, 1999). The most effective celebrity ads seem to be those that use a testimonial format, based on the celebrity's personal negative experiences with tobacco.

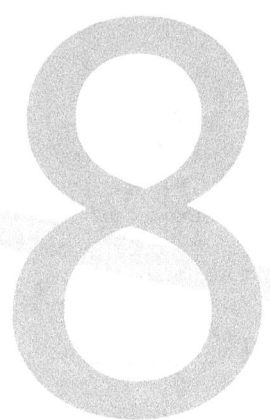

MESSAGE TONE, FREQUENCY, AND REACH

Message tone refers to the overall manner in which messages are delivered to and perceived by audiences. To a large extent, message tone is based on a number of perceived characteristics of message text and delivery. Message tone can have a strong impact on a viewer's reaction to an ad. Tone can also make ads emotionally draining and therefore difficult to continue watching.

Adequate media presence that ensures sufficient audience exposure to messages for substantial periods of time can be as important to ad effectiveness as the content and execution of the campaign's ads. Awareness of messages is often directly attributable to the media presence—a combination of the length of time ads are shown, the frequency of campaign messages, and the percentage of the target audience that they reach (Snyder, 2001).

Tobacco use prevention ads are aired in distinct cultural and media environmental contexts that can strongly influence their potential effects on audiences. For example, youth living in tobacco-growing communities may reject or ignore a tobacco counter-advertising message because smoking is an accepted behavior among their families and friends; in contrast, youth living in communities with strong tobacco control programs may have already been educated on the dangers of tobacco use and the industry's role in marketing tobacco products in ways that appeal to youth and therefore may be more inclined to accept anti-tobacco messages. As a result, the same messages could be received very differently by each audience.

How ads are executed (designed, edited, and produced) plays an important role in advertising effectiveness because potential effectiveness can be compromised by executing ads in ways that hinder communication or persuasiveness (Stevens, California Department of Health Services, oral communication, November 2000; Connolly, formerly of the Massachusetts Tobacco Control Program, oral communication, November 2000).

Humorous Versus Sad or Serious Tone

U.S./Utah

Formative research conducted by the Utah Department of Public Health showed that humorous ads got the attention of Utah youth, but these ads were not as persuasive as other ads tested with more serious and sad themes (Murphy, 2000).

U.S./Massachusetts

Researchers evaluated the role of message tone in U.S./Massachusetts anti-tobacco ads using the Massachusetts tobacco surveys. In 1997, 100 independent Massachusetts youth judges rated a group of anti-tobacco television ads for perceived effectiveness. The youth characterized the ads as sad or frightening (*Pam Laffin*, *Janet Sackman*, *Happy Birthday*, and *Cowboy*), funny (*Camel* and *Dinner*), or neutral (*Monica* and *Models*). The ads classified as sad or frightening were rated by the youth judges as more effective in causing them to think seriously about whether to smoke cigarettes than ads rated as funny or neutral (Biener, 2000). Some of the very sad and serious testimonial ads that aired in U.S./Massachusetts were perceived as too emotionally draining and therefore difficult to continue watching by some viewers (Brogdon, oral communication, October 2001).

U.S./Arizona

The Arizona prevention ads in-school evaluation tested the appeal and effect of emotion on the impact of anti-tobacco messages conveyed in ads aired in Arizona's youth-targeted tobacco counter-marketing campaign. The ads were rated for their ability to elicit emotional reactions. Ads rated as humorous, although well liked by youth, were perceived as less effective than other ads, especially those with more serious or sadder tones (Hendricks et al., 2001).

Preachy Tone

Scotland

Scottish youth reacted negatively to the tone actors used in the tobacco industry's European youth smoking prevention campaign. Describing the actors as "snobby," "bitchy," and "too perfect," participants in the Scotland MTV YSP Ads Focus Groups said that they found it difficult to identify with, and relate to, these ads (Devlin et al., 2002).

U.S./Florida and U.S./Minnesota

Programs in Florida and Minnesota, which featured industry deceptive-practices ads developed with the assistance of youth, found that ads needed to avoid "preaching" to audiences, telling youth how to think, feel, or act with respect to tobacco use (Ergo International, 2001; Sly, 1998). Because avoiding preachy messages was considered critically important to the Minnesota program managers, they included a measure of "preachiness" in the Target Market campaign evaluations. A quantitative study (a "brand audit") was designed to measure youth perceptions of the Target Market brand. The brand audit, conducted after the initial airing of Target Market ads, found that 46% of viewers who recalled the ads described them as "preachy," and this was considered a negative tone by youth (Ergo International, 2001). Program managers in Florida had a similar experience, reporting that ads featuring youth questioning authority became tiresome to youth audiences over time (Sly, 1998).

U.S./Mississippi and U.S./North Carolina

Formative message research by the Partnership for a Healthy Mississippi found that preachy messages are viewed cynically by youth (Partnership for a Healthy Mississippi, 2001). Youth focus-group participants warned the creative team that developed the tobacco use prevention ads in Mississippi against using a preachy tone in presenting tobacco information because this would cause them to ignore the message. As a result of these warnings, the Mississippi team developed ads conveying indisputable facts about tobacco that avoided telling viewers what to do. Researchers attending the University of North Carolina anti-smoking ads focus groups found that ads with adult-driven messages (e.g., featuring celebrities pitching a healthy lifestyle) were not viewed as credible by youth participants, partly because they contained an element of preachiness (University of North Carolina, 2001).

Although humorous ads may be appealing to youth, youth repeatedly rated ads as more effective in making them consider not smoking when the ads had a more serious or sad tone than when they had a humorous tone. This does not mean that ads with an ironic or sarcastic tone cannot be effective; these are common features of tobacco industry deceptive-practices ads. Ads with a preachy tone, especially those featuring adults telling youth what to do, should probably be avoided because youth audiences seem to especially dislike this tone.

Ad Frequency, Reach, and Duration

Mass media are the most efficient and effective means of reaching the youth audience (Zollo, 1999). Mass media generally include television, radio, print, direct mail, Internet, and billboard or other outdoor advertising. The mass media provide an important impetus for building awareness and understanding that helps other program elements effectively influence the target audience. Program developers have learned that using broadcast messages to increase awareness of tobacco issues can increase the impact of school- and community-based tobacco use prevention curricula (Flynn et al., 1995).

For example, U.S./Minnesota's youth tobacco use Target Market prevention program experienced a significant drop in awareness (from 85% to 57%) among youth aged 12–17 years surveyed just 6 months after annual funding was reduced from $23.7 million to $4.6 million in 2003, eliminating all broadcast presence (CDC, 2004). Over the same period, the percentage of adolescents susceptible to smoking (based on the number of friends and family members who smoke and the youths' attitudes toward tobacco and tobacco companies) increased from 43% to 53%.

Achieving media levels necessary to reach a large percentage of audiences with messages over long time periods is challenging. A meta-analysis of health campaigns in the United States found that, on average, only 40% of community-based intervention target audiences were exposed to the messages of these campaigns (Snyder, 2001). Insufficient media presence may explain why some large-scale experimental media campaigns have had little or no impact on behavior change (Hornik, 2002). Exposure to advertising needs to be sufficient to influence awareness, knowledge, attitudes, and behaviors. Even ads with strong and effective content that are delivered with an appropriate tone will not be effective unless a sufficient percentage of the target audience sees these ads regularly over a long period of time (Hornik, 2002).

A strong, consistent media presence is possible when media plans follow well-established industry guidelines developed over years of experience in evaluating media placement results for hundreds of products and services. These guidelines, which continually evolve over time as audience viewing habits change, are based on reach (estimated percentage of target audience exposed to ads), frequency (estimated number of times target audience members are exposed to the ads during a certain time period), and duration (length of time that a campaign continues to broadcast ads) of exposure.

Jeff McKenna, former Chief of the Health Communications Branch of CDC's Office on Smoking and Health for 12 years, developed recommendations regarding the reach, frequency, and duration of ads based on the scientific and advertising literature and CDC's experience in working with U.S. states and media experts on tobacco counter-marketing campaigns for adults and youth. Because these recommendations are based on experiences in the United States, they may not be applicable in all countries. The recommendations are:

- Ads should reach approximately 75%–85% of the target audience each quarter during the campaign.

- Managers should air ads as frequently as their budgets allow once this level of reach is achieved.

- Four-week target rating points (TRPs), which are the product of reach times frequency, should average 400 TRPs or more during the campaign's introductory phase and 200 TRPs or more after that. For example, if during the introductory phase 80% of the target audience is exposed to an ad an average of five times per 4-week period, the 4-week TRPs would be 400 (5 x 80), which should be sufficient.

- During the first 12 months of a campaign, ads should be aired as often as possible to establish the campaign themes and brand identity (if relevant).

- Ads should be aired for at least 6 months to affect awareness, 12–18 months to have an impact on attitudes, and 18–24 months to have an impact on behavior.

Note: A more in-depth discussion of guidelines for effective media planning can be found in *Advanced Calculations and Measurements, Advertising Media Planning* (Baron et al., 2002).

Tobacco companies spend billions of dollars on advertising each year, altering their marketing and advertising strategies and their messages in response to changing market conditions (Ling and Glantz, 2002). To counter the effects of this heavy marketing and to continue to influence target audience attitudes and behaviors over time, tobacco use prevention advertising must be continuously present in target audiences' minds.

Experienced media planners can provide valuable guidance in avoiding the pitfalls of spending too little money and reaping no benefit from messages heard sporadically by small numbers of people. In the case of extremely limited funds, program planners may need to pursue other interventions in addition to mass media, such as grassroots advocacy, to achieve desired environmental and policy changes.

Case histories showing the lessons learned from media campaigns in U.S./California, U.S./Massachusetts, and U.S./Florida, as well as a national U.S. campaign made possible through compliance with the Fairness Doctrine in the late 1960s and early 1970s, are included in Appendix 1. All of these campaigns involved a strong media presence over an extended period of time, and they are good examples of programs that changed attitudes and influenced behaviors, according to a variety of measures. Sufficient spending for ad placement and carefully developed creative messages contributed greatly to the success of these campaigns. When funding was reduced, limiting or eliminating media placement, campaign effectiveness was diminished (Balbach and Glantz, 1998; Abt Associates, 1999; Sly et al., 2002).

Ensuring sufficient audience exposure to messages may be as important as developing effective ads. Audiences must be exposed to messages enough times over long enough periods to be influenced by them. The results of research on tobacco counter-marketing campaigns support well-established media industry guidelines concerning the need to maintain a strong and consistent presence in broadcast media to achieve program goals. A long-term commitment to communicating counter-advertising messages through the mass media is essential to the long-term success of any campaign to prevent youth tobacco use.

Integration of Message Elements

Outstanding message content with high emotional appeal is not enough. Every aspect of an ad's development (format, tone, actors, setting, pace, etc.) must be done well. Airing several ads over the same time period, rather than just one ad (even one that has been found to be effective), is also essential to keep messages fresh and to prevent the ads from becoming so familiar to audiences that they do not pay attention to them (Stevens, California Department of Health Services, oral communication, November 2001; Connolly, Massachusetts Tobacco Control Program, oral communication, November 2001).

It is difficult, if not impossible, to distinguish the effects of each message element (content, format, tone) and environmental influence (Farrelly et al., 2003; Wakefield et al., 2003).

Two recent reviews of the scientific literature on media campaigns to prevent youth smoking highlight the need for further study of the many elements involved in creating an effective mass media campaign targeting youth. Farrelly et al. (2003) cited the need for research on the effects of message type, emotional content, and production values simultaneously to help determine precisely which campaign elements work most effectively to reduce smoking. These researchers pointed out the need to evaluate message effectiveness over time—messages currently known to be effective may wear out or only delay the onset of smoking. The review by Wakefield et al. (2003) shows that, although some campaigns have reduced smoking prevalence among youth, no single recipe appears to be the definitive approach.

These researchers suggest that inconsistent findings within and between campaigns may be due to the difference in methodologies, the fact that tobacco counter-advertising messages compete with many other broadcast messages for attention, the role of creative production factors, the extent of audience exposure to messages, message wear-out, and audience sophistication.

9 EVALUATION

Evaluation is critical to the effectiveness of tobacco control media campaigns (Atkin and Freimuth, 2001; Valente, 2002). But in too many cases, no evaluation is conducted, evaluation is done only as an afterthought, or evaluation is underfunded and thus not conducted properly or sufficiently. Tobacco control program managers need evaluation data to gauge whether campaign elements are being executed as planned and whether the target audience is seeing, hearing, and remembering the tobacco countermarketing messages. Evaluation is also needed to assess whether messages are affecting audience knowledge, attitudes, and beliefs, and ideally, whether the messages are contributing to behavior changes.

Evaluation must be planned from the beginning of any media campaign effort because it provides valuable information on how well campaign elements are being developed, how well the campaign is proceeding (while in progress), what the outcomes are over time, and whether changes to the campaign are needed. In addition, funders of tobacco counter-marketing campaigns generally require data to show that their funds were used to produce the desired effect. Without evaluation data, program planners will find it difficult to justify their tobacco counter-marketing activities.

The primary types of evaluation that should be included in media campaign planning include formative research and evaluation, process evaluation, and outcome evaluation. Examples of all three types of evaluation were reviewed in this document.

Formative research and evaluation are used to help develop advertising and other campaign materials. Formative research is typically qualitative and might include focus groups, observations, or one-on-one interviews. This type of research is used to discover key target audience insights that can be used to develop engaging and persuasive ad concepts. Once the ad concepts are developed, formative evaluation can be used to assess whether the proposed content, format, and tone of the ad concepts communicate the desired message clearly and persuasively to the target audiences. However, ads found to be successful in formative evaluation in one country or one region will not necessarily be successful elsewhere. (*Note:* Formative research and evaluation findings are reviewed under the "message research" sections of Chapter 6.)

Process evaluation helps managers determine whether a campaign's elements have been executed as planned. One typical use of process evaluation in a mass media campaign is to determine the level of audience exposure to ads during the period they were aired. Data from process evaluation are important not only for assessing exposure to ads, but also for identifying which ads are most or least remembered by, and compelling to, target audiences. This feedback can be used to make adjustments to certain ads or to the mix of ads used in the rest of the campaign.

For youth tobacco use prevention campaigns, process evaluation regarding the execution of the mass media placement plan is typically conducted in one of the following ways:

- Estimates of the size and makeup of the viewing audiences (often available from television and radio stations based on ratings for shows) and the number of times ads aired during a given period.

- Surveys of audience members, often by telephone, during or after an ad campaign to assess audience awareness of the ads. Typically, questions assess participants' potential level of exposure to ads, confirmed awareness of ads, and main message recall. Questions also address how engaging or persuasive the ads were to the viewers.

Outcome evaluation gauges changes in audience knowledge, attitudes, or intended or actual behavior. It is used to assess the effects of one ad or a whole campaign on a target audience. Achieving relevant outcome measures, such as increasing the percentage of the target audience that reports a strong commitment not to begin smoking or reducing the percentage of audience members reporting previous 30-day tobacco use, is the ultimate goal for many youth tobacco use prevention media campaigns.

Program managers recognize that outcome evaluations have some limitations. Behavior change at the population level is difficult to achieve over short periods of time and may not become evident for many months or years after a campaign begins. This underlines the need to continue to measure outcomes after a campaign ends. In addition, any observed behavior change cannot necessarily be attributed to a single tobacco control program element, such as a mass media advertising campaign.

ACKNOWLEDGMENTS

The authors wish to acknowledge the support and contributions of the tobacco control program managers and researchers in many countries, listed below, who so willingly provided their data and insights for this review. We thank Jeff McKenna, former Chief of the Health Communication Branch in the Office on Smoking and Health (OSH) at the Centers for Disease Control and Prevention, for his thoughtful insights and support. We also thank Terry Pechachek, PhD, Associate Director for Science at OSH, and Corinne Husten, MD, MPH, Acting Director of OSH, for their thoughtful comments and suggestions.

Jane Allen, MA/American Legacy Foundation, Washington, DC, USA

Eusebio M. Alvaro, PhD, MPH/Claremont Graduate University, Tucson, AZ, USA

Lois Biener, PhD/University of Massachusetts Boston, USA

Cindy Borgen/Minnesota Department of Health, St. Paul, USA

Mary Brogden/formerly with Arnold Communications, Boston, MA, USA

Greg Connolly, PhD, DDS/Harvard School of Public Health, Cambridge, MA, USA

Bill Coyne/Department of Health, London, England

Elinor Devlin/University of Strathclyde, Glasgow, Scotland

Matthew C. Farrelly, PhD/RTI International, Research Triangle Park, NC, USA

Kurt Fowler/Department of Health Services, Sacramento, CA, USA

Danielle Frissen/Defacto, The Hague, Netherlands

Stanton A. Glantz, PhD/University of California, San Francisco, USA

Anne Hafstad, PhD/National Institute of Public Health, Oslo, Norway

Kate Hassard/Anti-Cancer Council of Victoria, Canada

Natalie Lacey/Ipsos-Reid, Toronto, Canada

Anne Lavack, PhD/University of Regina, Canada

Mary Lee/Partnership for a Healthy Mississippi, Jackson, USA

Claudia Machado/Crispin Porter & Bogusky, Miami, FL, USA

Tim McGloin, MSPH/University of North Carolina at Chapel Hill, USA

Anne Miller/formerly with Arnold Communications, Boston, MA, USA

Cornelia Pechmann, PhD/University of California, Irvine, USA

Barbara Pizacani, PhD, MPH/Department of Human Services, Portland, OR, USA

Krzysztof Przewozniak, MA/Health Promotion Foundation, Warsaw, Poland

Kim Sanderson/Consultant with Many Hats, South Surrey, British Columbia, Canada

David F. Sly, PhD/University of Miami, FL, USA

Colleen Stevens, MSW/Department of Health Services, Sacramento, CA, USA

Paula Traffas/Texas Department of Health, Austin, USA

Melanie Wakefield, PhD/Centre for Behavioral Research in Cancer, Victoria, Canada

John K. Worden, PhD/University of Vermont, Burlington, USA

REFERENCES

Abt Associates, Inc. *Independent Evaluation of the Massachusetts Tobacco Control Program: Fifth Annual Report*. Boston: Abt Associates, Inc., Massachusetts Department of Public Health; 1999.

Abt Associates, Inc. *Independent Evaluation of the Massachusetts Tobacco Control Program: Sixth Annual Report*. Boston: Abt Associates, Inc., Massachusetts Department of Public Health; 2000.

Atkin C, Freimuth V. Formative evaluation research in campaign design. In: Rice RE, Atkin CK, editors. *Public Communication Campaigns*. 3rd edition. Thousand Oaks, CA: Sage; 2001:125–145.

Atkin C. Promising strategies for media health campaigns. In: Crano W, Burgoon M, editors. *Mass Media and Drug Prevention: Classic and Contemporary Theories and Research*. Mahwah, NJ: Lawrence Erlman; 2001:35–65.

Balch GI, Rudham G. Anti-smoking advertising campaigns for youth [letter]. *JAMA* 1998;280:323.

Balbach E, Glantz S. Tobacco control advocates must demand high-quality media campaigns: the California experience. *Tobacco Control* 1998;7:397–408.

Baron RB, Ephron E, Sissors JZ. *Advanced Measurements and Calculations in Advertising Media Planning*. 6th edition. New York: McGraw-Hill; 2002.

Bauer U, Johnson T. *Assessing the Impact of Florida's Pilot Program on Tobacco Control 1998 to 2000: A Comprehensive Analysis of Data from the Florida Youth Tobacco Survey*. Volume 3, Report 2. Tallahassee, FL: Florida Department of Health; 2001.

Bauer U, Johnson TM, Hopkins RS, Brook RG. Changes in youth cigarette use and intentions following implementation of a tobacco control program. Findings from the Florida Youth Tobacco Survey, 1998–2000. *JAMA* 2000;284:723–728.

Biener L. Adult and youth response to the Massachusetts anti-tobacco television campaign. *Journal of Public Health Management & Practice* 2000;6:40–44.

Biener L. Anti-tobacco ads by Massachusetts and Philip Morris: what teenagers think. *Tobacco Control* 2002;11(Suppl II):ii43–46.

Biener L, Harris JE, Hamilton W. Impact of the Massachusetts Tobacco Control Programme: population based trend analysis. *BMJ* 2000;321;351–354.

Biener L, Ji M, Gilpin E, Albers A. The impact of emotional tone, message and broadcast parameters in youth anti-smoking advertisements. *Journal of Health Communications* 2004;9:259–274.

Biener L, Taylor TM. The continuing importance of emotion in tobacco control media campaigns: a response to Hastings and MacFadyen. *Tobacco Control* 2002;11:75–77.

BMRB Social Research, COI Communications, Department of Health. *Tobacco Education Campaign Evaluation, Young People and Pregnant Smokers*. London: Department of Health; 2002.

British Columbia Ministry of Health. *Critics' Choice Post Analysis*. Victoria, BC; 2000.

Burgoon M, Miller C, Alvaro E, Denning V, Willey P, Grandpre J. Adolescents' responses to tobacco prevention TV ads. Poster presented at World Conference on Tobacco or Health; August 6–11, 2000; Chicago.

California Department of Health Services. *California Tobacco Control Update*. Sacramento, CA; 2000.

California Department of Health Services. *California Tobacco Control Update*. Sacramento, CA; 2002.

California Department of Health Services. *California Youth Tobacco Survey, 1994–2001*. Sacramento, CA; 2002.

Campaign for Tobacco Free Kids. *The Path to Smoking Starts at Very Young Ages*. Available at http://www.tobaccofreekids.org/research/factsheets/pdf/0127.pdf.

Centers for Disease Control and Prevention. *Best Practices for Comprehensive Tobacco Control Programs—August 1999*. Atlanta: U.S. Department of Health and Human Services; 1999.

Centers for Disease Control and Prevention. Effect of ending an antitobacco youth campaign on adolescent susceptibility to cigarette smoking—Minnesota, 2002–2003. MMWR 2004;53;301–303.

Centers for Disease Control and Prevention. *Preventing Tobacco Use Among Young People: A Report of the Surgeon General*. Atlanta: U.S. Department of Health and Human Services; 1994.

Centers for Disease Control and Prevention. Tobacco use among middle and high school students. US 2002. MMWR 2003;52:1096–1098.

Centers for Disease Control and Prevention. Youth tobacco surveillance summaries. MMWR 2001;50:1–84.

Devlin E, MacFadyen L, Hastings GB, Anderson S. Evaluation of the industry funded "Youth Smoking Prevention" (YSP) campaign. Presented at the 3rd European Conference on Tobacco or Health; June 20–22, 2002; Warsaw, Poland.

Dillard JP, Pfau M. *The Persuasion Handbook: Development in Theory and Practice*. Thousand Oaks, CA: Sage Publications; 2002.

Ergo International, Inc. *Target Market Campaign Evaluation: Pre-Post Research Results*. Minneapolis: Minnesota Partnership for Action Against Tobacco; 2001.

Farrelly MC, Davis KC, Haviland ML, Messeri P, Healton CG. Evidence of a dose-response relationship between "truth" antismoking ads and youth smoking prevalence. *American Journal of Public Health* 2005;95:425–431.

Farrelly MC, Davis KC, Yarsevich JM. Getting to the truth: assessing youths' reactions to the truth[sm] and Think. Don't Smoke. tobacco counter-marketing campaigns. *First Look Report 9*; 2002. Available at http://www.americanlegacy.org.

Farrelly MC, Niederdeppe J, Yarsevich J. Youth tobacco prevention mass media campaigns: past, present and future directions. *Tobacco Control* 2003;12(Suppl I):i35–47.

Flynn BS, Worden JK, Secker-Walker RH, Badger GJ, Geller BM. Cigarette smoking prevention effects of mass media and school interventions targeted to gender and age groups. *Journal of Health Education* 1995;26(Suppl):45–51.

Flynn BS, Worden JK, Selker-Walker RH, Pirie PL, Badger GJ, Carpenter JH, et al. Mass media and school interventions for cigarette smoking and prevention: effects 2 years after completion. *American Journal of Public Health* 1994;84:1148–1150.

Frissen D. DEFACTO for a smoke free future. Paper presented at Third European Conference on Tobacco or Health; June 19–21, 2002; Warsaw, Poland.

The Gallup Organization. *California Tobacco Control Prevention and Education Program: Waves 1, 2, 3 (1996–2000)*. Sacramento, CA: California Department of Health Services; 2003.

Glantz S. Changes in cigarette consumption, prices and tobacco industry revenues associated with California's Proposition 99. *Tobacco Control* 1993;2:311–314.

Goldman LK, Glantz SA. Evaluation of anti-smoking advertising campaigns. JAMA 1998;279:772–777.

Hafstad A, Aaro LE, Engeland A, Anderson A, Langmark F, Stray-Perersen B. Provocative appeals in anti-smoking mass media campaigns targeting adolescents—the accumulated effect of multiple exposures. *Health Education Research, Theory and Practice* 1998;12:227–236.

Hassard K, editor. *Australia's National Tobacco Campaign, Evaluation Report*. Volume 1. Canberra, Australia: Commonwealth Department of Health and Aged Care; 1999.

Hassard K, editor. *Australia's National Tobacco Campaign, Evaluation Report*. Volume 2. Canberra, Australia: Commonwealth Department of Health and Aged Care; 2000.

Hendricks A, Alvaro E, Burgoon M. Tobacco prevention and cessation: effectiveness of the Arizona Tobacco Education and Prevention Program. Presented at International Communication Association Annual Meeting; May 24–28, 2001; Washington DC.

Hopkins DP, Briss PA, Ricard CJ, Husten CG, Carande-Kulis VG, Fielding JE, et al. Reviews of evidence regarding interventions to reduce tobacco use and exposure to environmental tobacco smoke. *American Journal of Preventive Medicine* 2001;20(Suppl 2):16–66.

Hornik RC. Public health communication: making sense of contradictory evidence. In: Hornik RC, editor. *Public Health Communication: Evidence for Behavior Change*. Mahwah, NJ: Lawrence Erlbaum Associates; 2002;1–22.

Hu TW, Sung HY, Keeler TE. Reducing cigarette consumption in California: tobacco taxes vs. an anti-smoking media campaign. *American Journal of Public Health* 1995;85:1218–1222.

Independent Evaluation Consortium. *Final Report of the Independent Evaluation of the California Tobacco Control Prevention and Education Program*. Wave 1 data, 1996–1997. Rockville, MD: California Department of Health Services; 1998.

Institute of Medicine. *State Programs Can Reduce Tobacco Use*. A report of the National Cancer Policy Board. Washington, DC: National Research Council; 2000.

Johnson CA. Interviews with campaign designers/experts. In: Backer TM, Rogers EM, Sopory P, editors. *Designing Health Communications Campaigns: What Works?* Part 3. Thousand Oaks, CA: Sage Publications; 1992:113.

Lacey N, Ipsos-Reid. The Ontario experience. Presented at Tobacco Control Mass Media Round Table; July 8–9, 2002; Toronto, Ontario.

Lang A, Dhillon K, Dong O. The effects of emotional arousal and violence on television viewers' cognitive capacity and memory. *Journal of Broadcasting & Electronic Media* 1995;39;313–327.

Lantz PM. Smoking on the rise among young adults: implications for research and policy. *Tobacco Control* 2003;12(suppl 1):60–70.

Lavack A. *Canadian Anti-Tobacco Campaign: The Past Ten Years.* Regina, Saskatchewan: University of Regina; 2001.

Ling PM, Glantz S. Why and how the tobacco industry sells cigarettes to young adults: evidence from industry documents. *American Journal of Public Health* 2002;92:908–916.

Lewitt E, Coate D, Gorssman M. The effects of government regulation on teenage smoking. *Journal of Law and Economics* 1981;24:545–569.

Massachusetts Department of Health. *Ad Tracking Study.* Boston; 1997.

Massachusetts Department of Public Health. *Adolescent Tobacco Use in Massachusetts: Trends Among Public School Students, 1996–1999.* Boston; 2002.

Minnesota Department of Health. *Teens and Tobacco in Minnesota: Results from the Minnesota Youth Tobacco Survey.* Available at http://www.health.state.mn.us/divs/chs/data/youthtob.pdf.

Murphy RL. Development of a low budget tobacco prevention media campaign. *Journal of Public Health Management & Practice* 2000;6:45–48.

Murray DM, Prokhorov AV, Harty KC. Effects of a statewide anti-smoking campaign on mass media messages and smoking beliefs. *Preventive Medicine* 1994;23:54–60.

National Blueprint for Action. *Youth and Young Adults Tobacco Use Cessation.* Washington, DC: Center for the Advancement of Health for the Youth Tobacco Cessation Collaborative; 2000.

National Cancer Institute. Population based smoking cessation: proceedings of a conference on what works to influence cessation in the general population. *Smoking and Tobacco Control Monograph No. 12.* Bethesda, MD: U.S. Department of Health and Human Services, 2000. NIH Publication No. 00-4892.

Neiger BL, Barnes MD, Merrill RM, Murphy R, Thackeray R, Giles RT, et al. Measuring the effect of a tobacco media campaign among nonsmoking children and adolescents. *International Electronic Journal of Health Education* (serial online) 2002;5:35–40. Available at http://www.iejhe.org.

Partnership for a Healthy Mississippi. *2000 Ad Tracking Survey, Wave 4.* Jackson, MS: Southern Research Group, Mississippi State Department of Health, Mississippi State University Social Science Research Center; 2001.

Pechmann C, Zhao G, Goldberg ME, Reibling ET. What to convey in anti-smoking ads for adolescents? The use of protection motivation theory to identify effective message themes. *Journal of Marketing* 2003;67:1–18.

Petty RE, Cacioppo JT. *Communication and Persuasion: Central and Peripheral Routes to Attitude Change.* New York: Springer-Verlag; 1986.

Pierce JP, Gilpin EA, Emery SL, White MM, Rosbrook B, Berry CC, et al. Has the California tobacco control program reduced smoking? *JAMA* 1998;280:893–899.

Przewozniak K, Jaworski JM, Zatonski W. Counter-tobacco advertising campaign in Polish TV: approach and effects. Presented at Third European Conference on Tobacco and Health; June 19–22, 2002; Warsaw, Poland.

Puska P. The North Karelia Project: from community intervention to national activity in lowering cholesterol and CHD risk. *European Heart Journal* 1999;suppl 1:59–513.

Rogers RW. Cognitive and physiological process in fear appeals and attitude change: a revised theory of protection motivation. In: Cacioppo J, Petty R, editors. *Social Psychophysiology: A Source Book.* New York: Guilford Press; 1983:153–176.

Rothschild ML. *Marketing Communications.* Lexington, MA: D.C. Health & Co.; 1987.

RTI International. *Confirming the Truth: More Evidence of the Success of the Truth Strategy in Florida.* Results from the Legacy media tracking survey. Durham, NC; 2002.

Schar E, Gutierrez K. *A Review of Adult Cessation Media Campaigns in Nine Countries: World Health Organization—Tobacco Free Initiative.* Atlanta: U.S. Department of Health and Human Services, Centers for Disease Control and Prevention; 2001.

Slater MD. Entertainment education and the persuasive impact of narratives. In: Green MC, Strange JJ, Brock TC, editors. *Narrative Impact: Social and Cognitive Foundations.* Mahwah, NJ: Lawrence Erlbaum Associates; 2002:157–182.

Sly DF. *Florida Anti-Tobacco Media Evaluation, Report on September 1998 Survey Results.* Tallahassee, FL: Florida State University; 1998.

Sly DF, Heald G, Ray S. *Florida Anti-Tobacco Media Evaluation Follow Up Report*. Tallahassee, FL: Florida State University; 2001.

Sly DF, Trapido E, Ray S. Evidence of the dose effects of an anti-tobacco counter advertising campaign. *Preventive Medicine* 2002;53:511–518.

Sowden AJ, Arblaster L. Mass media interventions for preventing smoking in young people. *Cochrane Database of Systematic Reviews* 2003(1):CD001006.

Snyder L. How effective are mediated health campaigns? In: Rice R, Atkins C, editors. *Public Communication Campaigns*. 3rd edition. Thousand Oaks, CA: Sage Publications; 2001:181–190.

Task Force on Community Preventive Services. Review of evidence regarding interventions to reduce tobacco use and exposure to environmental tobacco smoke. *American Journal of Preventive Medicine* 2001;20(Suppl 1):10–15.

Teenage Research Unlimited. *Counter-Tobacco Advertising Exploratory, Summary Report*. Prepared for the States of Arizona, California, and Massachusetts Public Health Anti-Tobacco Media Campaigns. Northbrook, IL; 1999.

Terry-McElrath Y, Wakefield M, Ruel E, Balch GI, Emery S, Szczypka G, et al. The effect of anti-smoking advertisement executional characteristics on youth comprehension, appraisal, recall and engagement. *Journal of Health Communication* 2005;10:127–143.

Texas Tobacco Prevention Initiative. *Media Campaign and Community Program: Effects Among Children and Adults*. Austin, TX: University of Texas at Houston, Baylor College of Medicine, Texas Tobacco Prevention Initiative Research Consortium; 2001.

U.S. Department of Health and Human Services. *Preventing Tobacco Use Among Young People: A Report of the Surgeon General*. Atlanta: Centers for Disease Control and Prevention; 1994. U.S. Government Printing Office Publication No. S/N 017-001-00491-0.

U.S. Department of Health and Human Services. *Reducing the Health Consequences of Smoking: 25 Years of Progress. A Report of the Surgeon General*. Atlanta: Centers for Disease Control and Prevention; 1989.

U.S. Department of Health and Human Services. *Reducing Tobacco Use: A Report of the Surgeon General*. Atlanta: Centers for Disease Control and Prevention; 2000.

University of Arizona. *Evaluation of the TEPP Media Campaign*. Report 17, year 2, quarter 4: youth. Tucson, AZ; 2000.

University of Arizona. *Evaluation of the TEPP Media Campaign*. Report 29, year 4, quarter 1: youth comparisons. Tucson, AZ; 2002.

University of North Carolina at Chapel Hill. *Assessment of Anti-Tobacco Prevention Ads, Summary Statement 1999–2001*. Chapel Hill, NC; 2001.

Valente TW. *Evaluating Health Promotion/Health Communication Programs*. New York: Oxford University Press; 2002.

Wakefield M, Durrant R, Terry-McElrath Y, Ruel E, Balch G, Anderson S, et al. Appraisal of anti-smoking advertisements by youth at risk for regular smoking: a comparative study in the United States, Australia and Britain. *Tobacco Control* 2003;12(Suppl ii):ii82–ii86.

Wakefield M, Balch GI, Ruel EE, Terry-McElrath Y, Flay B, Szczypka G, et al. Youth appraisal of anti-smoking advertisements from tobacco control agencies, tobacco companies and pharmaceutical companies. *Journal of Applied Social Psychology* 2005;35:1899–1916.

Wakefield M, Flay B, Nichter M, Giovino G. Effects of anti-smoking advertising on youth smoking: a review. *Journal of Health Communications* 2003:8:229–247.

Warren CW, Jones NR, Eriksen MP, Asma S. Patterns of global tobacco use in young people and implications for future chronic disease burden in adults. *Lancet*. 2006;367(9512):749–753.

Worden JK, Flynn BS, Secker-Walker RH. Anti-smoking advertising campaigns for youth [letter]. JAMA 1998;280:323.

World Health Organization. *Tobacco Free Initiative*. Available at http://www.who.int/mediacentre/news/releases/2005/pr09/en/index.html.

Zollo P. *Wise Up to Teens: Insights into Marketing and Advertising to Teenagers*. 2nd edition. Ithaca, NY: New Strategist; 1999:155.

APPENDIX 1

CASE HISTORIES OF CAMPAIGNS WITH EFFECTIVE MEDIA PRESENCE

U.S./California

When Proposition 99 was enacted, funds were set aside for the development and implementation of a statewide tobacco counter-marketing campaign. The first wave of California's media campaign ran from April 1990 through September 1991 and cost $28 million. The media placement plan followed the generally recognized principles outlined in this report and achieved the recognized industry standards for media reach, frequency, and duration.

The California Tobacco Survey documented a 17% drop in the percentage of adults smoking during this period, which was attributed to the effects of a tax on tobacco products, educational efforts, and the media campaign (Balbach and Glantz, 1998). Before California's media campaign, cigarette consumption in the state had dropped by 45.9 million packs per year from 1981 to 1988. This rate of decline tripled to 164.3 million packs per year during the tobacco counter-advertising campaign, but decelerated to 19.4 million packs per year when the mass media portion of the campaign was withdrawn in 1992 (Balbach and Glantz, 1998).

A lawsuit by the American Lung Association restored funding for the media campaign from May 1992 through June 1993. The 1994–1995 budget was $12 million, but funding for the campaign was again reduced in 1995–1996, when only $6.5 million was spent. The reduced spending levels affected the intensity of the campaign, and the increase in adult smoking prevalence from 17.3% in 1994 to 18.4% in 1998 was attributed to the inadequate levels of media presence (Balbach and Glantz, 1998).

Per-capita spending on tobacco counter-advertising and promotions continued to decline in California from $5.73 in 1997–1998 to $3.42 in 1999–2000 (California Department of Health Services, 2002). During this period, overall smoking rates remained stable and media spending was below recommended CDC levels. At the same time, tobacco industry per-capita spending increased from $24.30 in 1997–1998 to $34.01 in 1999–2000 (California Department of Health Services, 2002).

Evaluators monitoring trends in California cigarette consumption and adult smoking prevalence from the early 1980s concluded that a substantial proportion of the decrease in cigarette consumption was attributable to the paid media campaign. The overall evaluation provides evidence that California's tobacco counter-marketing campaign was responsible for a substantial proportion of the observed declines in cigarette consumption and adult smoking behavior. The use of multiple data sources and evaluation approaches lends further support to this conclusion (Pierce et al., 1998; Glantz, 1993; Hu et al., 1995).

U.S./Massachusetts

The 1994–1998 Massachusetts tobacco control program budget averaged just under $40 million annually, with an annual media campaign budget of approximately $13 million in the initial launch period. The media budget declined to $11.09 million in 1999. Media placement planning followed the general guidelines provided in Chapter 8 of this report for reach, frequency, and duration, as recommended by the advertising agency of record, Arnold Communications. During this time, total per-capita cigarette purchases in Massachusetts declined by approximately

30%. Youth smoking prevalence declined slightly from 1995 to 1997 and the smoking rate among Massachusetts high school students declined again from 1997 to 1999, even though national rates were rising (Abt Associates, 1999).

U.S./Florida

The American Legacy Foundation's Media Tracking Survey results indicated that the more truth[sm] ads a youth viewed, the less likely he or she was to become a smoker. In the national tracking study, the Legacy Foundation surveyed Florida youth more frequently than youth in other states to fully examine the effect of their longer exposure to tobacco counter-advertising messages there, since Florida's Truth campaign had been conducted for several years before the national truth[sm] campaign was launched (RTI International, 2002).

Researchers evaluated the Florida Truth campaign by documenting the number of different ads that young respondents could describe. They found that the likelihood that a young nonsmoker would remain a nonsmoker increased with the number of Florida Truth anti-tobacco ads viewed. The researchers suggested that another valuable measure would be the number of times each ad had been viewed (Sly et al., 2002).

Although the Florida Truth campaign was adequately funded in its first year, it suffered funding cuts in subsequent years. During the well-funded year, smoking rates dropped 40% among middle school students and 18% among high school students. Once funding was cut, changes in smoking prevalence among youth leveled off. However, when the Legacy national truth[sm] campaign was launched (using a message focus similar to that of the Florida Truth campaign), it may have been able to compensate for the drop in Florida Truth campaign media levels (Sly et al., 2002).

U.S. Fairness Doctrine Campaign

A valuable field example of the power of sustained media campaigns is offered by the Fairness Doctrine campaign in the United States from 1967 to 1970. This campaign was the result of an agreement between the broadcast industry in the United States and the U.S. Federal Communications Commission, the agency that regulates the use of broadcast air waves. According to this agreement, the television networks were to donate placement of one anti-tobacco message as a public service announcement (PSA) for every three pro-tobacco ads paid for by the tobacco industry. As a result, sufficient levels of reach, frequency, and duration were achieved nationally for the first time to produce a high level of anti-tobacco message awareness.

The campaign was associated with declines in adult and teen smoking rates in the United States from 1968 to 1970 (U.S. Department of Health and Human Services, 1989). Smoking prevalence for all U.S. adults was 42.6% in 1966, the year prior to the Fairness Doctrine ruling, and had declined to 37.4% by 1970 when the PSAs ended. Per-capita cigarette consumption declined from 4,280 cigarettes in 1967 to 3,985 cigarettes in 1970, a relative decline of 7% (U.S. Department of Health and Human Services, 1989). During the period of anti-tobacco PSAs, teen-aged smoking declined by 3% (Lewit et al., 1981). Per-capita cigarette sales increased by 4% from 1971 to 1973 after the Fairness Doctrine PSAs ceased, rising from 3,985 to 4,148 cigarettes (U.S. Department of Health and Human Services, 1989).

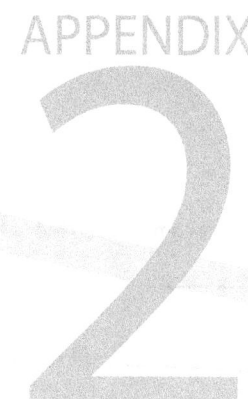

APPENDIX 2

LIST OF ADVERTISEMENTS BY COUNTRY AND U.S. STATE

Note: Some ads mentioned in this document were developed for research purposes only and were not part of an ongoing media campaign. These ads are listed under the relevant study in the research summary table (Appendix 3).

Australia

Campaign	*Every Cigarette Is Doing You Damage*
Origin Country	Australia, aired nationally
Sponsoring Organization	National Tobacco Campaign
Strategy/Objective	Motivate smokers to try to quit by: • Putting quitting on today's agenda. • Showing damage in a new way. • Tying damage to the act of smoking.
Primary Target	Smokers aged 18–40 years
Message	Every cigarette you smoke causes damage, so the sooner you quit, the better off you'll be.
Executions	Each spot is an empathetic portrayal of a slightly awkward but typical moment in the everyday life of a smoker. In some executions, the viewer journeys with cigarette smoke as it is inhaled, traveling down into the trachea and lungs, where the smoke begins its deadly work. In other executions, other facts are shared and other body parts are emphasized. • *Artery*—Fatty deposits, squeezed from the aorta. • *Lung*—Emphysematous damage. • *Tumour*—The recently discovered mechanism by which smoking damages the p53 tumor suppressor gene. • *Brain*—The mechanism of smoking-related strokes. • *Eye*—The impact smoking can have on eyesight and the fact that smoking is one of the leading causes of blindness. • *Tar Lung*—The amount of tar that collects in a smoker's lungs over time. • *Call for Help*—Cessation help line.
Elements	TV, radio, outdoor, print (including poster), and bus and tram ads; Web site www.quitnow.info.au; fold-out information sheets; launch events
Duration	June 1997–January 1999
Media Weights	1997—4 weeks at relatively high weights, followed by a 1-week break; 3 weeks on at medium levels with a 3-week break followed by 1 week on, 1 week off at low maintenance levels for 3 months 1998—Lower levels of TV advertising

APPENDIX 2   53

Canada/British Columbia

Campaign Name	***Critics' Choice Program*** (Ads produced in other countries were compared to the ad produced in Canada.)
Origin Country	Australia, British Columbia, Canada, U.S./American Legacy Foundation, U.S/Arizona, California, Massachusetts
Sponsoring Organization	British Columbia Ministry of Health
Strategy/Objective	Motivate youth to reject smoking by engaging them in discussion about anti-tobacco messages
Primary Target	Middle school and high school students
Message	The messages varied. For example, some ads focused on social consequences, some on stories of the impact of smoking on smokers and their families, and some on industry deceptive practices.
Executions	The executions tested or aired that are mentioned in this document are: • *Voicebox/Debi*—See description under U.S./California ads. • *Artery*—See description under Australia ads. • *Stroke*—See description under Australia ads. • *Tar Lung*—See description under Australia ads. • *Body Bags*—See description under U.S./American Legacy Foundation ads. • *Scary Math*—The number of Canadians affected by smoking-related illnesses.
Elements	In-school curriculum, TV
Duration	After the ads were tested in the Critics' Choice in-school program, one ad each year was selected to air in British Columbia. Durations of ad broadcasts are unknown.
Media Weights	Unknown

Canada/British Columbia

Campaign Name	***Protecting Kids from Tobacco***
Origin Country	British Columbia, Canada; U.S./California, Massachusetts
Strategy/Objective	Motivate adults and youth to reject tobacco
Primary Target	Primary target: Adults; Secondary target: Youth
Message	Smoking has consequences that cause pain and loss to both smokers and their loved ones.
Executions	Examples are listed below: • *Voicebox/Debi*—See description under U.S./California ads. • *Pam Laffin*—See description under U.S./Massachusetts ads. • *Janet Sackman*—See description under U.S./Massachusetts ads. • *Victor Crawford*—A former lobbyist for the tobacco industry says that tobacco companies target children because they know that 90% of smokers start as children. He then apologizes for his role, and the tag reveals that he died of throat cancer. • *Scary Math*—Discusses the number of British Columbians affected by tobacco-related illnesses.
Elements	In-school curriculum, youth advisory committee and network, Web site, TV ads, posters, magazine ads
Duration	June 1997–2001
Media Weights	Unknown

Canada/Ontario

Campaign Name	***Secondhand Smoke Educational Campaign*** (An ad produced outside Ontario was aired with ads produced in Ontario.)
Origin Country	Ontario, Canada
Sponsoring Organization	Ontario Ministry of Health (managed by Heart and Stroke Foundation and Ontario Lung Association)
Strategy/Objective	Educate the general public about the dangers of secondhand smoke to build support for clean indoor air policies
Primary Target	Adult voters and opinion leaders
Message	Secondhand smoke can endanger those you love and care about.
Executions	• *Victim/Wife*—See description under U.S./California ads. • *Don*—Description not available. • *Bernice*—Description not available.
Elements	TV, radio ads
Duration	April–July 2000 and December 2000–March 2001
Media Weights	Two TV flights lasting 16 weeks each

United Kingdom/England

Campaign Name	*Testimonials*
Origin Country	England
Strategy/Objective	Encourage smokers to quit by showing emotional pain of smokers and their families due to smoking-related illness and death
Primary Target	Adult smokers
Message	Smoking has consequences that cause pain and loss to both smokers and the non-smokers who care about them. The implied message is that smokers should quit. The ads were tagged with a toll-free quitline number.
Executions	Each execution was a real-life testimonial of a smoker or nonsmoker who had suffered from the consequences of smoking or losing someone to a smoking-related illness. • *Stephen*—A young man describes his illness caused by smoking. • *Rebecca*—A young woman describes the changes in her father due to his illness from smoking. • *Christy Turlington*—An American supermodel talks about losing her father to lung cancer 6 months after he quit smoking. She also shares how difficult it was for her to quit but views it as her biggest accomplishment. • *Byron, Colleen, Kay*—Testimonials. • *Pharmacist*—Asian chemist talks about using nicotine replacement therapy and refers the viewer to an undertaker standing nearby pointing out the alternative to not quitting, death. • *Relationships*—Family of smokers who have suffered smoking-related problems. • *Facts*—The number of people who die from smoking-related illnesses; provides quitline phone number.
Elements	TV, radio, and print ads
Duration	January–March 1998
Media Weights	Unknown

Finland

Campaign Name	*Youth-Targeted Campaign Within North Karelia Project*
Origin Country	Finland
Sponsoring Organization	National Public Health Institute
Strategy/Objective	Motivate youth to reject smoking by helping them resist social pressures to smoke
Primary Target	Youth
Message	You can quit too; you can resist smoking in social situations.
Executions	TV programming showing real-life experiences of North Karelians as they stopped smoking. School and community programs focused on building skills to resist smoking in social situations.
Elements	School and community-level programs, TV programming, adult cessation programs
Duration	1972–1997
Media Weights	7–15 TV shows over the years, 30–45 minutes each

The Netherlands

Campaign Name	*"…but I don't smoke."*
Origin Country	The Netherlands
Sponsoring Organization	*DEFACTO*
Strategy/Objective	Encourage youth to be nonsmokers by presenting nonsmokers in a positive light
Primary Target	Youth
Message	Nonsmokers can be cool, edgy, and rebellious. Young people do not need to smoke to be cool.
Executions	• *Restaurant*—Teenaged waiter, tired of requests for different items from older woman in restaurant, serves her urine in a glass. • *Classroom*—Teenaged boy burps in front of an entire classroom of students, including the teacher. • *Auto Shop*—Teenaged girls see auto mechanic working under a car and grab him in the crotch. • *Home*—Teenaged boy drinks milk directly from the carton and then punches his father when his father irritates him. • *Game Show*—Two teenaged girls spell names of genital organs and other sexually related words in a simulated game show. • *Bathroom*—Teenaged boy makes drunk, obnoxious man next to him in bathroom fall into urinal. • *Car*—Teenaged boy buys sexy women's underwear and places it in his father's car where his mother finds it and is horrified. Each execution ends with the teen saying, "…but I don't smoke."
Elements	TV ads
Duration	Unknown
Media Weights	Unknown

Norway

Campaign Name	*Provocative Appeals Campaign*
Origin Country	Norway
Sponsoring Organization	Cancer Registry of Norway; Research Center for Health Promotion, University of Bergen; Norwegian Women's Public Health Association
Strategy/Objective	Motivate youth, particularly girls, to reject smoking through provocative appeals
Primary Target	Teenaged girls (1992–1993); Teenaged boys and girls (1994)
Message	1992: Girls must be stupid because they know how bad smoking is for them but they still smoke. 1993: Smoking means lack of self-control and it conflicts with environmental concerns. 1994: Smoking means a lack of success in education and work.
Executions	One TV ad was produced and aired each year; print ads and posters were also developed.
Elements	TV, movie, and full-page newspaper ads; school posters
Duration	1992–1994
Media Weights	Each TV ad was aired 167 times over 3 weeks; each newspaper ad ran once in each of five newspapers; 1,140 posters were sent to schools and youth organizations each year.

Poland

Campaign Name	*Every Cigarette Is Doing You Damage*
Origin Country	Australia
Sponsoring Organization	Health Promotion Foundation
Strategy/Objective	Motivate smokers to try to quit by: • Putting quitting on today's agenda. • Showing damage in a new way. • Tying damage to the act of smoking.
Primary Target	Adult smokers
Message	Every cigarette you smoke causes damage, so the sooner you quit, the better off you'll be.
Executions	• *Artery*—See description under Australia ads. • *Stroke*—See description under Australia ads. • *Tar Lung*—See description under Australia ads. • *Brain*—See description under Australia ads.
Elements	TV ads and accompanying posters were part of comprehensive efforts related to the Quit and Win program, a promotion that encourages smokers to quit smoking and win prizes.
Duration	Unknown
Media Weights	Unknown

European Countries (38)

Campaign Name	*Youth Smoking Prevention Initiative*
Origin Country	Various European countries
Sponsoring Organization	British Tobacco, Japan Tobacco International, and Philip Morris
Strategy/Objective	Reduce youths' interest in smoking by showing them "cool" teens who do not smoke
Primary Target	Youth
Message	You can be cool and not smoke. You can have many interests other than smoking.
Executions	Each execution focuses on a teenager who has distinct interests but does not smoke. The copy says that he or she "does X, does Y, does Z, and doesn't smoke." The examples below are from Russia and Portugal: • *Silvia*—A teenage girl shops at a mall, trying on clothes, etc. • *Jaou*—A teenaged boy dances in clubs. • *Rodrigo*—A teenaged boy surfs. • *Katya*—A teenaged girl tries on clothes and then alters them to her own style. • *Lioha*—A teenaged boy plays in a rock band. • *Dimon*—A teenaged boy plays soccer.
Elements	TV ads
Duration	2001
Media Weights	Unknown. Aired in 38 European countries on the MTV network

U.S./American Legacy Foundation

Campaign Name	*truth*^sm
Origin Country	United States
Strategy/Objective	Motivate youth to reject smoking by providing information on the tobacco industry's deceptive marketing practices
Primary Target	Youth aged 12–17 years who are most at risk of smoking
Message	Messages vary by sub-campaign and execution, but the main messages are that tobacco companies make money by addicting youth to cigarettes, lying about the dangers of tobacco use, and manipulating the contents of cigarettes to make them more appealing while also making them more addictive and deadly.
Executions	Sample executions include: • *Body Bags* series—Body bags represent all of the people who die from smoking-related illnesses. The first and most famous execution shows teenagers unloading and piling up stacks of body bags in front of a tobacco company's headquarters while shouting that 1,200 people die every day from tobacco-related illnesses. The other executions show body bags on the beach, in bars, and on horseback to contrast the attractive images of smokers portrayed in cigarette ads with the reality of the death they cause. • *Daily Dose* series—Each execution focuses on one fact related to tobacco use or the behavior of the tobacco industry. In each ad, a teen holds up an electronic counter that lights up with the correct answer. • *Only One Product* series—Each ad portrays the typical use of a product; however, the third person to use the product in each ad is killed. The text reads that only one product kills one third of its users—tobacco.
Elements	TV and radio ads, Web site
Duration	Ongoing campaign that began in 2000
Media Weights	Ad-industry–recommended media weights to achieve awareness goals

U.S./Arizona

Campaign Name	*Tobacco Education and Prevention Campaign (TEPP)*
Origin Country	U.S./Arizona
Sponsoring Organization	Tobacco Education and Prevention Program, Arizona Department of Health Services
Strategy/Objective	Motivate youth to reject tobacco by showing disgusting and graphically intense tobacco-related images and situations in humorous ways to engage youth
Primary Target	Youth aged 14–18 years
Message	Although the messages varied throughout the many executions, the main message was that smoking is disgusting. A few notable exceptions include two ads about deciding whether to smoke, and one execution whose message is that tobacco does not always kill its users but it harms them in ways that may be just as bad.
Executions	Although executions vary greatly, each ad ends with the tagline, "Tobacco. Tumor-causing, teeth-staining, smelly, puking habit." Some sample executions are: • *Theater Snacks*—A boy and a girl are on a date in a movie theatre. He spits his chewing tobacco into his cup and then she takes his cup, drinks from it, and is horrified. • *Maggots*—A teenaged girl is preparing to go out and is smoking. As she continues to look in the mirror, her image turns into a witch and maggots come out of her mouth. • *I Decide*—Diverse teens state confidently that they decide what to do with their lives, they decide whether or not to smoke, and they choose not to smoke. • *Doesn't Kill*—Several teenagers say that tobacco did not kill their parents and friends as everyone thought it would. Then each parent or friend is shown and is clearly very ill.
Elements	TV, print, and radio ads; public relations events; Web site; merchandise
Duration	August 1998–2001
Media Weights	4-week flights airing periodically

U.S./California

Campaign Name	*California Tobacco Control Program*
Origin Country	U.S./California
Sponsoring Organization	California Department of Health Services, Tobacco Control Section
Strategy/Objective	De-normalize tobacco use by providing information about the tobacco industry's deceptive practices, health effects of tobacco use, dangers of secondhand smoke, and quitting resources
Primary Target	Adult smokers and nonsmokers
Message	Messages vary based on the themes stated above (industry deceptive practices, health effects of tobacco, health effects of secondhand smoke, quitting resources).
Executions	Examples of the many executions include: • *Voicebox/Debi*—A woman with a hole in her throat (stoma) tells her story of nicotine addiction. As she describes her unsuccessful attempts to quit, she inhales cigarette smoke through the stoma and questions the tobacco industry's unwillingness to admit that tobacco is addictive. The ad is tagged with the helpline phone number. • *Victim/Wife*—An older man recounts his wife's request that he quit smoking. Resentful of her interference, he had refused to quit, claiming that it was his life that was affected, not hers. In a broken voice, he explains that she died from the consequences of secondhand smoke. • *Hooked*—A fisherman dressed as a business executive is fishing. The voiceover discusses how the tobacco industry tries to "hook" youth with its addictive product. • *Quitting Takes Practice*—This animated spot depicts a sad and frustrated character who has tried unsuccessfully to quit smoking. The narrator points out that it took him a long time to start to smoke so it will probably take a more than a few tries to quit; quitting takes practice. By the end of the commercial, the smoker builds confidence in his ability to quit, using the helpline as a resource. The ad is tagged with the helpline phone number.
Elements	TV, radio, and print ads; billboards; public relations events
Duration	1988–1998
Media Weights	Minimum levels to achieve awareness goals and call volumes

U.S./Florida

Campaign Name	*Truth*
Origin Country	U.S./Florida
Sponsoring Organization	Florida Department of Health, Office of Tobacco Control
Strategy/Objective	Motivate youth to reject tobacco by informing them of deceptive tobacco industry practices
Primary Target	Youth aged 13–18 years
Message	Messages vary by execution; the main message is that the tobacco industry deceives people to make money from a deadly product.
Executions	Examples of the many executions include: • *Deaths Planned*—Simulating a motion picture trailer, this ad builds drama around a plot to kill millions of people and reveals at the end that it is the tobacco industry that is planning the deaths. • *Publishing*—An unscripted ad in which two teenaged boys call a magazine and ask why it accepts tobacco advertising, since the product kills. They then ask if the magazine would be willing to place anti-smoking ads for free. The magazine executive says "no" and hangs up. • *Director*—Two young men attempt to call a movie director to convince him not to have the characters in his film smoke. When one of the callers is unable to speak with the director personally, he leaves a detailed message with the secretary. • *Secrets*—Simulates an ad for a movie with scenes from the corporate life of a tobacco executive. This pseudo-movie trailer builds suspense and anticipation as the executive plots to gain the trust of young people to replace dying older cigarette smokers. • *Grim Reaper*—In a conference room filled with tobacco smoke, executives are discussing the profitability of filtered cigarettes. Suddenly, the Grim Reaper enters the room and complains that so many people are dying as a result of smoking that he cannot keep up with the workload. Eventually, security guards eject him from the room. • *Thanking Patient*—In a hospital room, a patient near death lies on a bed attached to a variety of medical devices. He is visited by two jovial tobacco executives who have come to thank him for his loyal business over the years, seemingly oblivious to the fact that the patient is in distress. When they notice a teenager in the hall who can replace the dying patient, the executives quickly approach her as if to begin the cycle over again. • *Fun with Statistics*—A laugh track plays in the background of actual footage of congressional hearings on the tobacco industry. This addition makes the testimony appear comical and embarrassing.
Elements	TV and print ads, billboards, public relations events, school curriculum
Duration	1998–2000
Media Weights	Unknown

U.S./Massachusetts

Campaign Name	*Massachusetts Tobacco Control Program*
Origin Country	U.S./Massachusetts
Sponsoring Organization	Massachusetts Department of Public Health
Strategy/Objective	De-normalize smoking by communicating new health-risk information about smoking and secondhand smoke, emphasizing the toll taken by tobacco-related illnesses on smokers and their families, providing quitting information, and exposing the deceptive marketing practices of the tobacco industry
Primary Target	Smokers; Secondary targets: youth, general population, and opinion leaders
Message	Messages varied based on the key themes, including health-risk information, impact on smokers and their families, cessation resources, and tobacco industry deceptive practices.
Executions	Examples of the many executions include: • *Pam Laffin Documentary* series—Pam speaks of the tremendous toll smoking has taken on her life. She started smoking at age 10 to look older. At age 24, she developed emphysema and had a lung removed. Individual executions focus on the pills that make her look bloated, the surgery, the failed lung transplant, the inability to breathe, her 20% chance of survival, and the impact on her children. • *Rick Stoddard* series—Rick talks about losing his wife (aged 46 years) to lung cancer caused by smoking. Each spot focuses on a different aspect of her illness, such as her addition to nicotine, her youth at the time of her death, and the pain she suffered as she died. • *Get Outraged* series—Each ad shows a previous disaster that concerned the U.S. public (e.g., poisoned grapes that killed a few people, a plane crash that killed hundreds of people), and then contrasts the reaction to these events to the relative lack of concern about tobacco, despite the fact that tobacco kills 1,200 people every day. The tag is, "Where is the outrage?" • *Youth Consequences* series—Each ad focuses on one negative consequence of smoking that is relevant to young people, such as wrinkles, high cost, compromised athletic performance, and social rejection, including by members of the opposite sex. • *Models*—Members of the U.S. women's soccer team talk about the advantages of not smoking, despite the messages from the tobacco industry that smoking will make a person glamorous or popular. • *Cowboy*—A man relates how his brother was one of the original Marlboro men in cigarette ads and how the tobacco companies wanted people to think that they could gain freedom and independence from smoking. The man's brother died of lung cancer from smoking. The man asks how someone can feel independent while hooked up to so many tubes and pieces of hospital equipment.
Elements	TV ads
Duration	Ongoing campaign began in January 1993. Evaluation results were reported through 2000. The *Pam Laffin* series ran for 11 weeks and the *Rick Stoddard* series ran for 7 weeks.
Media Weights	1,800 Gross Rating Points each for *Pam Laffin* and *Rick Stoddard* series

U.S./Minnesota

Campaign Name	*Target Market*
Origin Country	U.S./Minnesota
Sponsoring Organization	Minnesota Department of Health
Strategy/Objective	Motivate youth to reject tobacco by making them aware that tobacco companies target them with messages encouraging tobacco use
Primary Target	Youth aged 12–17 years
Message	Tobacco companies are targeting us, so let's target them by uncovering and rejecting their marketing practices.
Executions	Sample executions are below: • *Thank You*—Individual teens speak to the camera, saying "thank you" to the tobacco industry in a sarcastic voice for convincing kids to smoke, killing family members, deceiving people about their products, and other acts. • *Light It Up*—Youth construct a giant cowboy out of tobacco ads ripped from magazines (meant to symbolize the Marlboro Man) and burn it, while the voiceover says that tobacco companies still spend millions of dollars on ads in the magazines that youth read. • *Bigger Than Ever*—Teenagers rip up all of the tobacco ads they can find in magazines and create a sign that reads, "They're Still Targeting Us."
Elements	TV, print, and radio ads
Duration	2000–July 2003
Media Weights	Unknown

U.S./Mississippi

Campaign Name	*Question It*
Origin Country	U.S./Mississippi
Sponsoring Organization	Partnership for a Healthy Mississippi
Strategy/Objective	Motivate youth to reject tobacco by providing information about the deceptive marketing practices of the tobacco industry and facts about the health risks of smoking
Primary Target	Youth (smokers and nonsmokers) aged 12–18 years
Message	Messages vary by execution and include the following themes: tobacco industry deceptive marketing practices, the role addiction plays in new-customer acquisition, dangers of tobacco use compared with other negative life experiences, and short-term health effects.
Executions	Sample executions include: • *Cheerleader*—A cheerleader coughs and drops a fellow cheerleader in a cheering competition. • *Car Contest*—An endurance contest for a car is lost by a teenager who coughs just as the opposition is weakening. • *Barber*—A teenaged boy sits in a barber chair for a haircut. The barber gives him a comb-over hair style, mimicking the style used for older men waiting in the room. The voiceover asks, "You wouldn't want their haircut, why would you want their lungs?" • *Dentist*—A teenaged girl in the dentist's chair has all of her teeth removed and replaced with diseased-looking teeth. The voiceover says, "You wouldn't want their teeth, why would you want their lungs?" • *License*—A strutting teenager receives his driver's license and backs his car into a patrol car as he exits the parking lot. A voiceover says, "That's one way screw up your life early. Smoking is another." • *Cow-tipping*—Teenagers playing pranks tip over cows in the field, but one cow tips over on top of a kid. The voiceover says, "That's one way screw up your life early. Smoking is another." • *Prisoner*—A prisoner is being led to the electric chair as the voiceover describes how many people he has killed. At the end, it is revealed that the "killer" is a tobacco industry executive. • *It's Legal*—The head drug dealer tells a group of street-wise drug dealers that it is time to focus on a drug that is just as addictive as other drugs but is easier to push because it is legal—tobacco. All of the ads end with the tagline, "Question It."
Elements	TV, radio, and outdoor ads; contests; Web-based reality programs; school curriculum; public relations events; posters
Duration	Ongoing campaign that began in March 1999
Media Weights	Unknown

U.S./Mississippi

Campaign Name	*Reject All Tobacco (R.A.T.)*
Origin Country	U.S./Mississippi
Sponsoring Organization	Partnership for a Healthy Mississippi
Strategy/Objective	Motivate youth to reject tobacco by teaching them about the health effects of smoking and secondhand smoke; empower them to speak up to adults to protect themselves from secondhand smoke and promote quitting in those they care about
Primary Target	Youth aged 6–11 years
Message	Smoking is dangerous to smokers and nonsmokers. Make sure you tell someone about it.
Executions	Humorous presentations of the dangers of tobacco use and secondhand smoke to youth and adults in their lives, including: • *Goldfish*—A woman's pet fish shows its love for her by blowing bubbles in the form of hearts and then extinguishes her cigarette, while the voiceover admonishes the audience to tell someone to quit smoking today so that they will be around tomorrow. • *Robot*—A scientist training a robot to show emotion is surprised when the robot cares enough to take a cigarette out of his mouth. A voiceover tells the audience to help someone quit smoking today so that they will be around tomorrow. • *Fly*—A fly attempts to escape the dangers of secondhand smoke from the cigarette of a woman driving with her daughter in the car. A voiceover talks about the number of toxic chemicals in secondhand smoke. • *X-Ray Goggles*—A boy with x-ray glasses sees the insides of his father's lungs, which are filled with tar from smoking. The voiceover discusses the number of deaths from cancer due to smoking. • *Aunt Edna*—A young boy experiences a vivid dream in which a bizarre aunt becomes responsible for his care after the death of his parents from smoking-related diseases. The next morning the boy sees his parents prepare to smoke at the breakfast table and tells them to quit smoking so they will be around in the future. • *Foosball*—A foosball game begins and the cigarette smoke from the boys playing the game makes the players sick. The voiceover describes the health effects of secondhand smoke, such as lung cancer, asthma attacks, and reduced physical performance. • *Toy Soldier*—Animated toy soldiers mourn the loss of the toy soldier who was smoking a cigarette; the voiceover points out that 4 million people a year die from smoking-related illnesses around the world.
Elements	TV, radio, and outdoor ads; contests; Web site; performance troupe; school curriculum; public relations events; posters; merchandise
Duration	Ongoing campaign that began in May 1999
Media Weights	Unknown

U.S./Oregon

Campaign Name	*Tobacco Use Prevention Program*
Origin Country	Ads were produced by U.S./California and U.S./Massachusetts and aired in U.S./Oregon
Sponsoring Organization	Tobacco Control Program, Oregon Department of Health
Strategy/Objective	Motivate smokers to try to quit
Primary Target	Smokers
Message	Message varied by ad execution, but most focused on the pain and suffering smokers and their family members suffered because of smoking-related illnesses and death.
Executions	• *Voicebox/Debi*—See description under U.S./California ads. • *Cowboy*—See description under U.S./Massachusetts ads. • *Pam Laffin*—See description under U.S./Massachusetts ads. • *Janet Sackman*—See description under U.S./Massachusetts ads. • *Victim/Wife*—See description under U.S./California ads.
Elements	TV ads
Duration	Unknown
Media Weights	Unknown

U.S./Philip Morris

Campaign Name	*Think. Don't Smoke.*
Origin Country	United States
Strategy/Objective	Motivate youth to reject smoking by giving them the choice about whether to smoke
Primary Target	Youth aged 10–14 years Secondary target: Parents of youth aged 10–14 years
Message	You can decide whether to smoke, and you don't have to smoke to be cool or popular. In addition, some ads focused on the short-term health effects of smoking on athletic performance.
Executions	The campaign included many executions; those mentioned in this document are: • *Bus*—An African American teenaged boy says that he does not want to smoke and that it is stupid. • *Stairs*—Racially diverse teens talk about their decisions not to smoke. • *Karate Kid*—A preteen in a karate class finds that smoking affects endurance.
Elements	Primarily TV ads
Duration	2000–2002
Media Weights	Unknown

U.S./Texas

Campaign Name	*Tobacco Is Foul*
Origin Country	U.S./Texas
Strategy/Objective	Motivate youth to reject tobacco
Primary Target	Youth aged 11–12 years
Message	Short-term health effects
Executions	• *Gotta Light*—An animated character introduces a smoker who desperately needs to light a cigarette. An athlete carrying a torch runs by and the smoking character runs to catch the flame. He is not able to catch the runner because of his smoke-damaged lungs. • *First-Time Smokers*—Two animated characters try smoking an abandoned cigarette butt they discover on the playground. Inhaling the smoke causes them to choke and gag. An x-ray of their lungs shows the impact of smoking on their ability to breathe. The first-time smokers decide that smoking is not for them. • *Tobacco Show Off*—An animated character sets up a fight between animated characters who are chewing and smoking tobacco. The fighters collapse from weakness due to smoking and the grossness of chewing tobacco.
Elements	TV ads, school and community prevention programs, and adult cessation programs
Duration	Spring–Fall 2000
Media Weights	Unknown

U.S./Utah

Campaign Name	*The Truth About Tobacco*
Origin Country	U.S./Utah
Sponsoring Organization	Utah Department of Health
Strategy/Objective	Motivate youth to reject tobacco by exposing the myths about the positive aspects of smoking
Primary Target	Youth
Message	Many myths are out there. Find out the truth about smoking by calling a toll-free phone number.
Executions	Sample executions include: • *Pam Laffin*—See description under U.S./Massachusetts ads. • *Janet Sackman*—See description under U.S./Massachusetts ads. • *Voicebox/Debi*—See description under U.S./California ads. • *Cowboy*—See description under U.S./Massachusetts ads. • *Negative Role Models*—Utah teenagers at the Great Salt Lake explain why they started smoking. • *Positive Role Models*—Utah teenagers at various Utah locations explain why they do not smoke.
Elements	TV, radio, magazine, and newspaper ads; school programs
Duration	Ongoing campaign that began in 1998
Media Weights	Unknown

U.S./Vermont, New York, Montana

Campaign Name	*University of Vermont Northeastern States Study*
Origin Country	U.S./Vermont
Sponsoring Organization	University of Vermont
Strategy/Objective	Motivate youth to reject tobacco by providing such information as the negative social consequences of smoking and the positive social consequences of not smoking, and refusal skills
Primary Target	Youth
Message	Executions focused on the negative social consequences of smoking, positive social consequences of not smoking, short-term and long-term health effects of smoking, cost of smoking, and how to refuse an offered cigarette.
Executions	Examples of the many executions include: • *Beautiful Lady*—An attractive woman enjoying an evening of leisure experiences wrinkled skin, discolored teeth, and other effects of smoking. • *Billy*—A young boy encourages his friends to smoke with him, but is repeatedly rebuffed by those who think that smoking is wrong, including his dog. • *Don't Worry*—Teenagers discover that they can perform better at singing, swimming, and other pursuits than competitors who smoke. • *Break Away*—Teens enjoy the positive aspects of not smoking, encouraged to "break away" by a rock band performing the song "Breakaway." • *Nicoflame*—An animated segment features a young boy learning about the short-term and long-term consequences of smoking—dizziness, bad breath, yellow teeth, tar in lungs, and high blood pressure. The voiceover encourages him to say, "No, I don't smoke." • *Drag Race*—An animated segment introduces the addictive aspects of smoking and encourages youth to say, "No, I don't smoke." • *Viewpoints of Ex-Smokers*—Ex-smokers offer testimonials about the additive nature and short-term health effects of smoking. • *Viewpoints of Nonsmokers*—Nonsmokers share testimonials about the health effects and costs of smoking, and reasons not to smoke.
Elements	TV ads, school curriculum
Duration	January–April 1986–1989
Media Weights	Average annual paid media presence over 4-month period was 190 spots on network TV and 350 spots on cable TV in each market. Media outlets also donated public service airtime, increasing the number of broadcasts up to 50%.

APPENDIX 3
RESEARCH SUMMARY

APPENDIX 3

Study	Common Name	Research Sponsor	Methods	Ads Involved
Australia National Tobacco Campaign Surveys[1]	Australia National Tobacco Campaign Surveys	Commonwealth Department of Health and Family Services	Smokers and recent quitters aged 18–40 years (n = 1,979): pre-campaign May 1997 (n = 2,981): post-campaign November 1997 Telephone surveys	Lung, Artery, Tumour
Australia South Australian Health Omnibus Survey 1997[1]	South Australian Health Omnibus Survey 1997	South Australian Smoking and Health Project	Youth and adults aged 15 years and older (n = 3,019) 15–17 years (n = 160) 18–40 years (n = 1,300) 41+ years (n = 1,559) Face-to-face interviews in participants' homes	Ads from Stressing Out—You're Smarter Than That campaign (ads unknown) "Every Cigarette Is Doing You Damage": Lung, Artery, Tumour
Canada National Tobacco Use Monitoring Survey 1996, 1997, 1999, 2000, 2001	Canadian Tobacco Use Monitoring Survey	Health Canada National Population Health Survey	Youth aged 15–19 years (n = 3,087) Telephone surveys	Unknown
Canada/British Columbia Critics' Choice[2] 1997, 1998, 1999, 2000	Critics' Choice School Program	British Columbia Ministry of Health	Elementary, middle, and secondary schools, classroom voting after viewing 12 anti-tobacco ads *Number of Participants by Year* 1997 22,000 1998 43,275 1999 65,025 2000 60,000	**1997**—*Voice Box, Pee Pee, Janet Sackman, Ice, Dinner, Pam Laffin, Victor, Scary Math, Joy, Cattle, Attractiveness, Mosh Pit* **1998**—*Aorta, Maggot, Christy, Ashes, Cigar, Tumour, Date, Smoke, Mascot, I Decide, Truth, Subliminal, Spoiled* **1999**—*Stroke, Cocktail, Best Memory, Joanne, Can't Breathe, Airplane, Talk Show, Tea Party, Scary Math, Grasshopper, War, Cowboy* **2000**—*Tar, Body Bags, Eye, Breathe, Splode, Ironic Quotes, Theater Snacks, Rid-A-Zit, Fish Out of Water, Parachute, Larc, Voice*

[1] Hassard K, editor. *Australia's National Tobacco Campaign, Evaluation Report.* Volume 1. Canberra: Commonwealth Department of Health and Aged Care; 1999.

[2] British Columbia Ministry of Health. *Critics' Choice Post Analysis.* Victoria, BC; 2000.

Study	Common Name	Research Sponsor	Methods	Ads Involved
Canada/Ontario Ontario Tobacco Media Campaign Tracking Survey—Youth 2001	Ontario Tobacco Media Campaign Tracking Survey—Youth	Ontario Provincial Government	Youth (n = 305) Adults (n = 1,000) Telephone survey	*Beautiful Lady, Billy, Breakaway, Don't Worry, Drag Race, Jennifer, Magazine Ad, Mindy, Nicoflame, Older Girl, VP Ex-Smokers, VP Nonsmokers*
England Anti-Smoking Advertising Tracking, Survey Wave 6[3]	Anti-Smoking Advertising Tracking Survey	Central Office of Information, on behalf of the Department of Health, England; BMRB Social Research	Youth aged 11–15 years (n = 301) Face-to-face interviews	*Stephen, Rebecca, Christy, Kay, Byron, Colleen, Pharmacist, Relationship, Facts*
Finland National FINRISK Study[4] 1972, 1977, 1982, 1987, 1992, 1997	North Karelia Project	Department of Epidemiology and Health Promotion, National Public Health Institute, Helsinki	Men aged 30–59 years (n = 19,761) Women aged 30–59 years (n = 20,761) Surveys to assess cardiovascular disease risk following a comprehensive community-based intervention initiated in 1972 to reduce coronary heart disease mortality rate in 35- to 64-year-old males	Messages were primarily delivered through TV programming
International Global Youth Tobacco Survey 2002	Global Youth Tobacco Survey	Centers for Disease Control and Prevention; World Health Organization	Students aged 13–15 years 75 sites in 43 countries and the Gaza Strip/West Bank School-based survey	No ad evaluation

[3] BMRB Social Research, COI Communications, Department of Health. *Tobacco Education Campaign Evaluation, Young People and Pregnant Smokers.* London: Department of Health; 2002.

[4] Puska P. The North Karelia Project: from community intervention to national activity in lowering cholesterol and CHD risk. *European Heart Journal* 1999;suppl 1:59–513.

APPENDIX 3

Study	Common Name	Research Sponsor	Methods	Ads Involved
International Youth Appraisal of Anti-Smoking Advertising 2000, 2001[5,6,7]	NCI Youth Appraisal of Anti-Smoking Advertising	State and Community Tobacco Control Initiative of the National Cancer Institute	Youth smokers or susceptible nonsmokers (n = 615) • U.S. grades 8, 10, or 12 (n = 278) • Australia grades 8, 10, or 12 (n = 162) • United Kingdom British equivalent to grades 8, 10, or 12 (n = 157) Participants viewed and evaluated 10 ads. A follow-up phone call 1 week later evaluated recall and engagement.	50 ads representing a range of messages produced by tobacco control agencies (37), tobacco companies (8), and pharmaceutical companies (5)
Netherlands The DEFACTO Tracking Study 1998–2001	Netherlands DEFACTO Tracking Study	DEFACTO	Youth aged 12–16 years (n = 600)	"…but I don't smoke." campaign (see Appendix 2 for descriptions of ads)
Norway Provocative Appeals in Adolescent-Targeted Mass Media Campaigns, 1992 and 1995[8]	Norway Youth Provocative Appeals Campaign Evaluation	Cancer Registry of Norway; Institute for Epidemiological Cancer Research, Oslo; Research Center for Health Promotion, University of Bergen; Norwegian Women's Public Health Association	Adolescents aged 14 and 15 years in intervention county (n = 4,898) Adolescents aged 14 and 15 years in control county (n = 5,439) Survey questionnaire completed in classrooms	Ads unknown Main message was that girls must be stupid because they know the risks of smoking and still smoke

[5] Wakefield M, Durrant R, Terry-McElrath Y, Ruel E, Balch G, Anderson S, et al. Appraisal of anti-smoking advertisements by youth at risk for regular smoking: a comparative study in the United States, Australia and Britain. *Tobacco Control* 2003;12(Suppl ii):ii82–ii86.

[6] Wakefield M, Balch GI, Ruel EE, Terry-McElrath Y, Flay B, Szczypka G, et al. Youth appraisal of anti-smoking advertisements from tobacco control agencies, tobacco companies and pharmaceutical companies. *Journal of Applied Social Psychology* 2005;35:1899–1916.

[7] Terry-McElrath Y, Wakefield M, Ruel E, Balch GI, Emery S, Sczypka G, et al. The effect of anti-smoking advertisement executional characteristics on youth comprehension, appraisal, recall and engagement. *Journal of Health Communication* 2005;10:127–143.

[8] Hafstad A, Aaro LE, Engeland A, Anderson A, Langmark F, Stray-Petersen B. Provocative appeals in anti-smoking mass media campaigns targeting adolescents—the accumulated effect of multiple exposures. *Health Education Research, Theory and Practice* 1998;12:227–236.

Study	Common Name	Research Sponsor	Methods	Ads Involved
Poland Evaluation of 1999–2001 Media Campaigns	Poland Media Campaign Evaluation	Great Polish Smokeout Campaign	Youth aged 13–15 years (n = 3,294) Youth aged 16 years (n = 1,100) Telemetric Measurement System by Centre of Research on Public Opinion	Great Polish Smokeout Campaign, using the Every Cigarette Is Doing You Damage campaign ads
Poland Poland (Urban) Global Youth Tobacco Survey 1999	Poland (Urban) Global Youth Tobacco Survey	Centers for Disease Control and Prevention; World Health Organization	Youth aged 13–15 years (n = 1,576) School-based survey	Ads unknown
Scotland Evaluation of Tobacco Industry-Funded MTV Youth Smoking Prevention Campaign—Focus Groups, 2001	Tobacco Industry-Funded MTV Youth Smoking Prevention Campaign—Scotland Focus Groups	University of Strathclyde	Youth aged 12–17 years Eight focus groups	Main message of campaign was, "You can be cool and not smoke" (see Appendix 2 for descriptions of ads)
U.S./Arizona Evaluation of the Tobacco Education and Prevention Program Media Campaign[9]	Arizona Tobacco Education and Prevention Program Media Campaign Evaluations	Communication Research Section, Arizona Cancer Center, University of Arizona	Smokers and nonsmokers aged 11–17 years (n = 853) Telephone surveys	*Chuck's Mom, Doesn't Kill*, Truth ad series 1–5 (see Appendix 2 for descriptions of ad series)
U.S./Arizona Evaluation of the Tobacco Education and Prevention Program Media Campaign[10]	Arizona Tobacco Education and Prevention Program Media Campaign Evaluations	Communication Research Section, Arizona Cancer Center, University of Arizona	Youth aged 11–17 years (n = 308) Exposure and recall rates Telephone surveys Compared data from 1998 and 2001	Media schedule was not active during this period. Recall measures were for national truth[sm] spots, *Ammonia, Rat Suit,* and *BioSphere*.

[9] University of Arizona. *Evaluation of the TEPP Media Campaign.* Report 17, year 2, quarter 4: youth. Tucson, AZ; 2000.

[10] University of Arizona. *Evaluation of the TEPP Media Campaign.* Report 29, year 4, quarter 1: youth comparisons. Tucson, AZ; 2002.

APPENDIX 3

Study	Common Name	Research Sponsor	Methods	Ads Involved
U.S./Arizona Impact of Prevention Ads on Tobacco Attitudes and Intentions[11]	Arizona Prevention Ads In-School Evaluation	Arizona Cancer Center, University of Arizona	Students in grades 6–12 (n = 1,831) In-school survey	*Theater Snack, Maggots, Grasshopper, Bucking Bronco, Smoked Meat, I Would Rather, Rapunzel, Frank, Pee Pee, Mosh Pit, Rodeo Rider, Basketball, Lady Bug, Runner, I Decide*
U.S./California Protection Motivation Theory Message Testing[12] 1998, 2000	Protection Motivation Theory Message Study, University of California, Irvine	California Tobacco-Related Disease Research Program, University of California, Irvine	7th-grade students (n = 788) 10th-grade students (n = 879) Participants completed a written survey after viewing a videotape of eight ads in a classroom setting	The 56 ads tested were randomly selected from among 194 compiled from all known English-language sponsors of anti-smoking ads and represented the themes of disease and death, endangerment of others, cosmetic effects, smokers' negative life circumstances, refusal-skills role models, marketing tactics, selling disease and death
U.S./California Independent Evaluation Consortium[13] 1996–1997, 1998, 1999–2000	California Gallup Independent Evaluation Consortium	Gallup Organization; Stanford University; University of Southern California	Adults from 18 focal counties (n = 6,916) Telephone interviews Students from 18 focal counties (n = 26,479) School-based surveys	A broad range of ads with messages about health risks, tobacco industry deceptive practices, secondhand smoke, and cessation resources

[11] Burgoon M, Miller C, Alvaro E, Denning V, Willey P, Grandpre J. Adolescents' responses to tobacco prevention TV ads. Poster presented at World Conference on Tobacco or Health; August 6–11, 2000; Chicago, IL.

[12] Pechmann C, Zhao G, Goldberg ME, Reibling ET. What to convey in anti-smoking ads for adolescents? The use of protection motivation theory to identify effective message themes. *Journal of Marketing* 2003;67:1-18.

[13] Independent Evaluation Consortium. *Final Report of the Independent Evaluation of the California Tobacco Control Prevention and Education Program. Wave 1 data, 1996–1997.* Rockville, MD: California Department of Health Services; 1998.

Study	Common Name	Research Sponsor	Methods	Ads Involved
U.S./California California Tobacco Surveys (CTS) 1990–1991, 1992, 1993, 1996, 1999, and 2002. In addition to the 1996 basic CTS survey, a 1993–1996 Teen Longitudinal Survey was released.	California Tobacco Surveys	The California Department of Health Services contracted with the University of California, San Diego; Westat Corp.	Surveys of attitudes, behaviors, and media exposure regarding smoking and tobacco use	Evaluated recall of all program elements, including televisions ads presenting health risk, tobacco industry deceptive practices, secondhand smoke, and cessation messages
U.S./Florida Anti-Tobacco Media Evaluation[14,15,16] 1998, 1999, 2000	Florida Anti-Tobacco Media Evaluation	Center for the Study of Population, College of Social Sciences, Florida State University	Youth aged 12–20 years (n = 2,110) Telephone surveys conducted every 6 months between October 1998 and October 2000	Broad variety with focus on messages about tobacco industry deceptive practices, including *Director, Producer, Publishing, Who Are You, Congrats, Agency, Vending, That's the Problem, Lucky, Lungs, I'm an Actor*
U.S./Florida Youth Tobacco Survey 1998, 1999, 2000[17,18]	Florida Youth Tobacco Survey	Bureau of Epidemiology, Florida Department of Health	Public middle school (grades 6–8) and high school (grades 9–12) students Self-administered school-based surveys Year Gr 6–8 Gr 9–12 # schools 1998 11,865 10,675 242 1999 11,724 9,254 242 2000 13,961 9,784 243	Broad variety, primarily with messages about tobacco industry deceptive practices

[14] Sly DF. *Florida Anti-Tobacco Media Evaluation, Report on September 1998 Survey Results*. Tallahassee, FL: Florida State University; 1998.

[15] Sly DF, Heald G, Ray S. *Florida Anti-Tobacco Media Evaluation Follow Up Report*. Tallahassee, FL: Florida State University; 2001.

[16] Sly DF, Trapido E, Ray S. Evidence of the dose effects of an anti-tobacco counter advertising campaign. *Preventive Medicine* 2002;53:511–518.

[17] Bauer U, Johnson T. *Assessing the Impact of Florida's Pilot Program on Tobacco Control 1998–2000: A Comprehensive Analysis of Data from the Florida Youth Tobacco Survey*. Volume 3, Report 2. Tallahassee, FL: Florida Department of Health; 2001.

[18] Bauer U, Johnson TM, Hopkins RS, Brook RG. Changes in youth cigarette use and intentions following implementation of a tobacco control program. Findings from the Florida Youth Tobacco Survey, 1998–2000. *JAMA* 2000;284:723–728.

APPENDIX 3

Study	Common Name	Research Sponsor	Methods	Ads Involved
U.S./Massachusetts Department of Public Health Advertising Tracking Study 1997	Massachusetts Ad Tracking Study 1997	Arnold Communications; Millersville University Opinion Research Center	Students from Massachusetts (n = 600) and New Hampshire (n = 300) 25 female, 25 male respondents per grade per cell Quasi-quantitative tracking study via in-school interviews among students aged 11–14 years (grades 5–7)	*Pam Laffin* and *Break Free* campaigns
U.S./Massachusetts Tobacco Suveys in 1993, 1996, 1999[19,20,21,22,23,24]	Massachusetts Tobacco Surveys	Center for Survey Research, University of Massachusetts, Boston	Adults in 1993 (n = 1,500) Re-interview of participants in 1996 Youth aged 14–17 years (n = 733) Random-digit–dialed telephone survey in 1999, identified in earlier adult survey process Telephone survey Behavioral Risk Factor Surveillance System data Tobacco Institute Reports	Teen panels assigned ads to the following categories: 1. Massachusetts ads depicting illness, in which people told their stories about health consequences of smoking and loss 2. Massachusetts *Get Outraged* campaign, a series of messages about deaths caused by tobacco and the tobacco industry's targeting of youth 3. Massachusetts ads that focused on sports performance, social acceptance, and being cool, with no mention of health consequences 4. Philip Morris's *Think, Don't Smoke.* youth campaign, which communicated that youth are free to choose whether to smoke

[19] Biener L. Adult and youth response to the Massachusetts anti-tobacco television campaign. *Journal of Public Health Management & Practice* 2000;6:40–44.

[20] Biener L. Anti-tobacco ads by Massachusetts and Philip Morris: what teenagers think. *Tobacco Control* 2002;11(Suppl II):ii43–46.

[21] Biener L, Harris JE, Hamilton W. Impact of the Massachusetts Tobacco Control Programme: population based trend analysis. *BMJ* 2000;321;351-354.

[22] Biener L, Ji M, Gilpin E, Albers A. The impact of emotional tone, message and broadcast parameters in youth anti-smoking advertisements. *Journal of Health Communications* 2004;9:259–274.

[23] Biener L, Taylor TM. The continuing importance of emotion in tobacco control media campaigns: a response to Hastings and MacFadyen. *Tobacco Control* 2002;11:75–77.

[24] Massachusetts Department of Public Health. *Adolescent Tobacco Use in Massachusetts: Trends Among Public School Students, 1996–1999.* Boston; 2002.

Study	Common Name	Research Sponsor	Methods	Ads Involved
U.S./Minnesota Minnesota-Wisconsin Adolescent Tobacco Use Research Project	Minnesota-Wisconsin Adolescent Tobacco Use Research Project	University of Minnesota; Minnesota Department of Health; National Research Centre for Preventive Medicine, Moscow, Russia	9th-grade students (n = 3,900) surveyed annually in 43–46 community units roughly equivalent to school areas	Variety of ads with themes of social disapproval of smoking due to negative social consequences of tobacco use, bad breath and smelly clothes, and social approval of nonsmoking
U.S./Minnesota Target Market Campaign Evaluation Pre/Post Research Results 2000, 2002, 2003, 2004[25]	Minnesota Target Market Campaign Evaluations	Minnesota Department of Health; Survey Research Center, University of Florida	Youth aged 12–17 years (n = 1,000) Telephone survey	Variety of ads, primarily with theme of tobacco industry deceptive practices (see Appendix 2 for descriptions of selected ads)
U.S./Minnesota Minnesota Youth Tobacco Survey 2000, 2002[26]	Minnesota Youth Tobacco Survey	Minnesota Department of Health	Students in grades 6–12 in 101 middle and high schools (n = 11,557)	No ad evaluation
U.S./Mississippi Mississippi Youth Benchmark Study Ad Tracking Survey Wave 4 2001[27]	Mississippi Youth Ad Tracking Benchmark Survey	Partnership for a Healthy Mississippi; Southern Research Group	Students in grades 3–12 Cell phone survey conducted at schools (n = 1,510)	**Reject All Tobacco ads:** *Aunt Edna, Barber, Bingo, Car Contest, Cheerleader, Cow Tipping, Fly, Foosball, Frances, Goldfish, License, Prisoner PHM, Robot, Teeth, Toy Soldier, VJ, X-Ray Goggles* **Question It ads:** *Cheerleader, Car Contest, Barber, Dentist, License, Cow-Tipping, Prisoner PHM, It's Legal*

[25] Ergo International, Inc. *Target Market Campaign Evaluation: Pre-Post Research Results*. Minneapolis: Minnesota Partnership for Action Against Tobacco; 2001.

[26] Minnesota Department of Health. *Teens and Tobacco in Minnesota: Results from the Minnesota Youth Tobacco Survey*. Available at http://www.health.state.mn.us/divs/hpcd/tpc/TobaccoReports.html.

[27] Partnership for a Healthy Mississippi. *2000 Ad Tracking Survey, Wave 4*. Jackson, MS: Southern Research Group, Mississippi State Department of Health, Mississippi State University Social Science Research Center; 2001.

APPENDIX 3

Study	Common Name	Research Sponsor	Methods	Ads Involved
U.S./Mississippi Youth Behavior Risk Survey 1991, 1993, 1995-1997	Mississippi Youth Behavior Risk Surveys	Division of Adolescent and School Health, Centers for Disease Control and Prevention	Students in grades 9-12 (n = approximately 1,500 annually) Self-administered questionnaire	No ad evaluation
U.S./Mississippi Youth Behavior Risk Survey Middle Schools 2003	Mississippi Youth Behavior Risk Survey of Middle Schools	Mississippi State Department of Health	Students in grades 6-8 (n = 1,510) Self-administered in-school questionnaire	No ad evaluation
U.S./Mississippi Youth Risk Behavioral Survey 2001	Mississippi Youth Risk Behavioral Survey 2001	Mississippi State Department of Health	Middle school students in 34 schools (n = 1,500)	No ad evaluation
U.S./Mississippi Youth Tobacco Survey, 1998	Mississippi Youth Tobacco Survey	Mississippi State Department of Health	Students in grades 6-12 Self-administered school-based survey Public high school students (n = 1,710) Private high school students (n = 1,537) Middle school students (n = 1,725)	No ad evaluation
U.S./Multistate Meta-Analysis of Health Campaigns[28]	Meta-analysis of 48 health campaigns	University of Connecticut	Total (n = 168,147) Meta-analysis of 48 health communication campaigns in the United States promoting a wide range of health behaviors Campaigns included at least one form of mass media and were community-based	No ad evaluation
U.S./Multistate Literature Review of Youth Tobacco Use Prevention Media Campaigns[29] 2002	Literature Review of Youth Tobacco Use Prevention Media Campaigns	Research Triangle Institute	Literature review of youth tobacco use prevention mass media campaigns	No ad evaluation

[28] Snyder L. How effective are mediated health campaigns? In: Rice R, Atkins C, editors. *Public Communication Campaigns*. 3rd edition. Thousand Oaks, CA: Sage Publications; 2001:181–190.

[29] Farrelly MC, Niederdeppe J, Yarsevich J. Youth tobacco prevention mass media campaigns: past, present and future directions. *Tobacco Control* 2003;12(Suppl I):i35–47.

Study	Common Name	Research Sponsor	Methods	Ads Involved
U.S./Multistate Teen Research Unlimited Focus Groups[30]	Teen Research Unlimited Multi-State Focus Groups	State health departments in Arizona, California, and Massachusetts; Centers for Disease Control and Prevention	At-risk youth aged 12–16 years (n = 120) 20 focus groups in six cities in three states	*Pam Laffin, Cowboy, Voicebox/Debi, Industry Spokesman, I Decide, Pee Pee, Publishing, Cinema: Deaths Planned, Bus, Stairs*
U.S./National Legacy Media Tracking Surveys[31,32]	Legacy Media Tracking Surveys	American Legacy Foundation	Youth aged 12–17 years Young adults aged 18–24 years Pre-campaign (n = 6,897) 10 months after campaign started (n = 10,692) Telephone surveys	Variety of ads including the American Legacy Foundation's *Body Bags* and several ads from the Philip Morris Think. Don't Smoke. campaign (see Appendix 2 for descriptions of individual ads)
U.S./National Quantitative Copy Testing 1997	National Quantitative Copy Testing	Centers for Disease Control and Prevention	Youth aged 13–19 years (n = 98) ARS quantitative copy testing in eight U.S. cities	*Cowboy/Will McLean, Models*
U.S./National Evaluation of Anti-Smoking Advertising Campaigns Focus Group Analysis 1998	National Anti-Smoking Campaign Focus Group Analysis	University of California, San Francisco	Youth and adults (n = 1,500) 186 focus groups	118 ads produced for California, Massachusetts, and Michigan tobacco counter-advertising campaigns
U.S./National National Youth Tobacco Survey 2002	National Youth Tobacco Survey	American Legacy Foundation	Middle school students (n = 12,581) High school students (n = 13,358) School-based survey	No ad evaluation
U.S./North Carolina Focus Groups 2001	North Carolina Anti-Smoking Ads Focus Groups	University of North Carolina	Youth aged 12–15 years (n = 91) 10 focus groups	*Pam Laffin, Lab Monkey, Injuries, Rick Stoddard* series—*Heart in the Sky; Target Market* series—*Thank You;* American Legacy Foundation truth[sm] series—*Barrio Marketing, Venus, Gwen, Ribbons, 1 in 3, 2nd Hand*

[30] Teenage Research Unlimited. *Counter-Tobacco Advertising Exploratory, Summary Report.* Prepared for the States of Arizona, California, and Massachusetts Public Health Anti-Tobacco Media Campaigns. Northbrook, IL; 1999.

[31] Farrelly MC, Davis KC, Yarsevich JM. Getting to the truth: assessing youths' reactions to the truth[sm] and Think. Don't Smoke. tobacco counter-marketing campaigns. *First Look Report 9*; 2002. Available at http://www.americanlegacy.org.

[32] RTI International. *Confirming the Truth: More Evidence of the Success of the Truth Strategy in Florida. Results from the Legacy media tracking survey.* Durham, NC: 2002. Available at http://tobacco.rti.org/data/lmts.cfm.

APPENDIX 3

Study	Common Name	Research Sponsor	Methods	Ads Involved
U.S./North Carolina Anti-Smoking Ads Focus Groups 2000	North Carolina Anti-Smoking Ads Focus Groups	University of North Carolina at Chapel Hill	Youth aged 12–16 years Four focus groups	*Pam Laffin, Cowboy, Voicebox/Debi, Industry Spokesman, I Decide, Pee Pee, Publishing, Cinema: Deaths Planned, Bus, Stairs*
U.S./Utah Tobacco Prevention Media Campaign Formative Message Research[33]	Utah Tobacco Media Campaign Formative Message Research	Utah Department of Health	Youth aged 11–18 years (n = 285) Theater testing of 35 radio and TV ads Eight focus groups throughout Utah	Participants identified top 10 preferred ads focusing on prevention from pool of 35 ads: *Voice Box/Debi, Cowboy, Bad Influence, Janet Sackman, Cattle, Pam Laffin, Smart Dog, Movie, Camel, Girlfriend, Maggots*
U.S./Utah Tobacco Prevention Media Campaign Evaluation[34]	Utah Tobacco Media Campaign Evaluation	Utah Department of Health	Nonsmokers aged 9–18 years (n = 596) Telephone surveys before and after the campaign	*Pam Laffin, Janet Sackman, Cowboy, Debi/Voicebox, Teenagers at Great Salt Lake, Teenagers Why I Don't Smoke, The Truth About Tobacco*
U.S./Vermont Multistate School and Mass Media Combination Interventions[35]	Multistate School and Mass Media Campaign Combination Evaluations	University of Vermont	Students in grades 5–7 (n = 5,458) initially Students in grades 10–12 (n = 5,458) by end of campaign Six in-school surveys in four matched study communities in Vermont, New York, and Montana	Broad range of ads (see Appendix 2, Vermont for descriptions of selected ads)

[33] Murphy RL. Development of a low budget prevention media campaign. *Journal of Public Health Management & Practice* 2000;6:45–48.

[34] Neiger BL, Barnes MD, Merrill RM, Murphy R, Thackeray R, Giles RT, et al. Measuring the effect of a tobacco media campaign among nonsmoking children and adolescents. *International Electronic Journal of Health Education* (serial online) 2002;5:35–40. Available at http://www.iejhe.org.

[35] Flynn BS, Worden JK, Secker-Walker RH, Badger GJ, Geller BM. Cigarette smoking prevention effects of mass media and school interventions targeted to gender and age groups. *Journal of Health Education* 1995;26(Suppl):45–51.

| U.S./Vermont
Mass Media and School Interventions for Cigarette Smoking Prevention Follow-Up[36] | Multistate Mass Media and School Interventions Follow-Up | University of Vermont | Students in grades 10–12 (n = 4,670) assessed in the 1986–1990 cigarette smoking prevention study
Primary outcome was cigarette smoking in the past week | 36 television ads developed and produced by six creative agencies in several formats: situation comedy, rock video, cartoon, testimonial, and drama. Spots included *Beautiful Lady, Billy, Don't Worry, Break Away, Nicoflame, Drag Race,* and *View Points* (see Appendix 2 for descriptions of individual ads) |

[36] Flynn BS, Worden JK, Selker-Walker RH, Pirie PL, Badger GJ, Carpenter JH, et al. Mass media and school interventions for cigarette smoking and prevention: effects 2 years after completion. *American Journal of Public Health* 1994;84:1148–1150.